T0202411

The Ethics of Uncertainty

The Ethics
of Uncertainty

*Entangled Ethical and Epistemic Risks
in Disorders of Consciousness*

L. SYD M JOHNSON

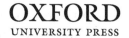

OXFORD
UNIVERSITY PRESS

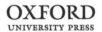

OXFORD
UNIVERSITY PRESS

Oxford University Press is a department of the University of Oxford. It furthers
the University's objective of excellence in research, scholarship, and education
by publishing worldwide. Oxford is a registered trade mark of Oxford University
Press in the UK and certain other countries.

Published in the United States of America by Oxford University Press
198 Madison Avenue, New York, NY 10016, United States of America.

Library of Congress Cataloging-in-Publication Data
Names: Johnson, L. Syd M., author.
Title: The ethics of uncertainty : entangled ethical and epistemic risks in
disorders of consciousness / L. Syd M Johnson.
Description: New York : Oxford University Press, [2022] |
Includes bibliographical references and index. |
Identifiers: LCCN 2021031199 (print) | LCCN 2021031200 (ebook) |
ISBN 9780190943646 (hardback) | ISBN 9780190943677 (epub) | ISBN 9780190943653
Subjects: MESH: Consciousness Disorders |
Uncertainty | Risk Management—ethics
Classification: LCC R724 (print) | LCC R724 (ebook) | NLM WL 341 |
DDC 174.2—dc23
LC record available at https://lccn.loc.gov/2021031199
LC ebook record available at https://lccn.loc.gov/2021031200

DOI: 10.1093/med/9780190943646.001.0001

1 3 5 7 9 8 6 4 2

Printed by Integrated Books International, United States of America

The Poems of Emily Dickinson: Variorum Edition, edited by Ralph W. Franklin, Cambridge,
Mass.: The Belknap Press of Harvard University Press, Copyright © 1998 by the President and
Fellows of Harvard College. Copyright © 1951, 1955 by the President and Fellows of Harvard
College. Copyright © renewed 1979, 1983 by the President and Fellows of Harvard College.
Copyright © 1914, 1918, 1919, 1924, 1929, 1930, 1932, 1935, 1937, 1942 by Martha Dickinson
Bianchi. Copyright © 1952, 1957, 1958, 1963, 1965 by Mary L. Hampson.

For Zoë and Izzy,
and for Mal, who lived and died while I wrote this.

I felt a Cleaving in my Mind –
As if my Brain had split –
I tried to match it – Seam by Seam –
But could not make them fit –

The thought behind, I strove to join
Unto the thought before –
But Sequence ravelled out of Sound –
Like Balls – upon a Floor –

—Emily Dickinson (1896)

Contents

Preface

This book is primarily about two things. One is disorders of consciousness (DoCs). The other is epistemic and ethical uncertainty, how they interact, and how they might be managed in a way that helps us in thinking about, and making decisions for, patients with DoCs. DoCs are an important case study for what I call the ethics of uncertainty, but they are also what inspired this, an approach to ethics that acknowledges and wrestles with uncertainty. Bioethics should be grounded in reality. It should be down to earth, where there's mud to get stuck in, where we risk getting our hands dirty. It should, if we do it right, increase tension and hold it, confront uncertainty and its implications. This is a work of applied ethics, and particularly, bioethics. I expect and hope that the ethical approach I propose in these pages will have broader applications and implications, beyond DoCs.

Part of what prompted this book, the focus on DoCs, and the embrace of the tensions (from multiple directions and dimensions) is the disorders themselves, their unique history, and their unique place at the center of a number of formative debates in academic bioethics, clinical medicine, and the public sphere. DoCs and especially the "vegetative state" are familiar to people who have no particular and abiding interests in medicine or bioethics. They've heard of the vegetative state (or more likely, the outdated but still widely used term "persistent vegetative state"). They've thought about it, and think they have pretty settled views on what they think about it, and what they would want themselves, should they ever be someone in a vegetative state. I was one of those people for a good chunk of my life. I remember vividly when I was a child and

Karen Ann Quinlan's legal case was front page news. I accepted the orthodox view that those in a vegetative state were hopeless cases whose lives were without meaning, purpose, or value.

A curious thing happened. In 2009, a case involving a patient named Rom Houben, in Belgium, generated international headlines. Houben had been diagnosed as being in a vegetative state, and he remained that way for two decades, but he was suddenly able to communicate using a method called facilitated communication, in which a therapist helps an individual move their hands across a board or touchscreen, allowing them to form words and sentences. Houben was said to be writing a novel. He reportedly poignantly said of his years of forced silence "I screamed, but there was nothing to hear." Steven Laureys, a neurologist and researcher at Belgium's Coma Science Group, reported that Houben's metabolic brain function, as revealed by a positron emission tomography (PET) scan, was nearly normal.

It turned out to be a hoax, although perhaps not an intentional one. Facilitated communication is widely discredited—the facilitators can, intentionally or not, exercise too much control over what the patient "says" by guiding their hands. Houben's facilitator later acknowledged that she had unwittingly done that.[1] But the curious case prompted me to look again at DoCs and to appreciate for the first time the unsettling fact of their high rates of misdiagnosis. It was a time of great upheaval, even without hoaxes, when a number of unsettling and remarkable discoveries were being made about DoCs and DoC patients, including research on patients who could "respond" to commands by controlling their brain activity. Renewed scientific and bioethical interest in DoCs followed.

Two related things prompted me to write this book. One is that a lot of what has been written about the ethics of DoCs is now out of

---

[1] Laureys, the neurologist, tested Houben again, this time showing him objects when the facilitator was not present. Later, Houben (and his facilitator) could not answer simple questions about the objects.

date and out of touch with the facts as we know them today. (Those facts may change tomorrow.) The second is that although I'm trained as a philosopher, and I know that bioethics, like philosophy, can be done from an armchair, I think a lot of the philosophizing and bioethicizing that has been done about DoCs over the last several decades has been too abstract, from too remote an armchair, if you will. When you write about DoCs, you may think you're writing about an abstract patient, but you are also writing about real patients, real people *in extremis*, and they have families and friends who care about them. Thought experiments may be about people, but people are not thought experiments. So, I had concerns about some of the conclusions that had been reached, conclusions about whether DoC patients were persons, or humans, or alive, about whether they mattered morally.

I'm interested in the uncertainty of DoCs and its epistemic and ethical implications. But I am also interested in how teasing apart the entangled uncertainties might help us be better epistemic and moral agents as we wrestle with complex questions related to patients like those with DoCs. The attentive reader will find that, by the end of this book, the uncertainties remain (they might be worse, if I've done my job), and that the definitive answers and ethical pronouncements made by others have been shown to be problematic and unsupportable. In other words, the reader looking for a clear-cut answer to the general question *What should we do about, and for, DoC patients?* will not find it. I hope in the end the reader will share my doubts about both the possibility of answering that question and the propriety of asking it.

This book is divided into three parts of three chapters each. Chapters 1, 2, and 3 deal with some preliminaries that are needed to set up the arguments made in the three chapters in part II—arguments for an ethics of uncertainty that uniquely addresses the kinds of epistemic and ethical uncertainty that plague our thinking and decision-making about DoCs and DoC patients. Part III looks at some persistent puzzles and applications of the ethics of uncertainty.

Chapter 1 provides a brief sketch of some theories of consciousness, particularly those that have some explanatory use in thinking about DoCs, as well as those that are revisited in later chapters. There is no pretense that chapter 1 provides anything approaching a complete account of all the questions, problems, or theories of consciousness. The important point for our purposes is that we don't know what consciousness is, which hinders efforts to detect it in nonparadigmatic cases. Chapter 2 is a selective account of the history of DoCs, and how epistemic and ethical certainty about what was initially known as the persistent vegetative state gradually gave way to ethical and ontological *un*certainty, partly as a function of scientific and clinical progress that led to greater appreciation of the epistemic uncertainty of these disorders. In Chapter 3, the way the pieces connect begins to surface. The problem of misdiagnosis and how it affects patients—how neglect of the physical, emotional, and psychosocial needs of patients is harmful—are illustrated by the vivid experiences and words of Kate Bainbridge, one of the first documented patients with cognitive motor dissociation. Confusion about consciousness, or types or modes of consciousness—between global and local states of consciousness—contributes to the misdiagnosis problem, as does the mismatch between what is being looked *for* and what is being looked *at* in a diagnosis of consciousness.

In the second part of the book, the distinctive form and focus of the ethics of uncertainty take shape. Chapter 4 examines the kinds of inferences that are common in the diagnosis and prognosis of DoCs. I develop an application of the concept of inductive risk— the epistemic risk of being wrong—to the inferential uncertainties that beset us in the diagnosis and prognosis of DoCs. To respond to inductive risk, I propose two principles of inductive risk that index epistemic risks to ethical risks. In chapter 5, my concern is with the decisions made by surrogates and healthcare staff, and with risk inversion. Risk inversion occurs when greater, certain, immediate risks are undertaken to prevent lesser or merely speculative future risks. I refer to these as upstream and downstream risks in the context of DoCs, because the uncertain risks exist downstream, in the future, while potential solutions lie upstream. Withdrawing treatment shortly after a brain injury, when a patient is comatose, results in the death of the patient—that's the upstream risk. The speculative downstream risk is that the patient will survive but would wish that they had not. Inverting those risks means undertaking a certain risk in order to avoid an uncertain risk. In chapter 6, I assemble the pieces into the ethics of uncertainty. The ethics of uncertainty is meant to be sensitive and responsive to the epistemic uncertainty that comes with ethical risks, and to the intersections where epistemic and ethical uncertainty interact. Central to this approach to ethics are considerations of justice. In bioethics, justice has frequently been limited to thinking about distributive justice, or the just allocation of medical and healthcare resources. DoC patients have frequently been targeted in that distribution, with their continued care deemed wasteful or futile. I reject using healthcare as a distributive scalpel and instead turn my focus to epistemic justice, and *epistemic* distributive justice, as well as the demanding duties of epistemic agents (particularly physicians and other medical staff).

The third part turns to some questions and applications related to consciousness and the ethics of uncertainty. Chapter 7 aims to show why consciousness is not a suitable criterion for determining who is, and who is not, a person with moral status. I am skeptical that there are defensible, necessary, nonmoral criteria for a moral property like "personhood" or "moral status." But assuming there are such criteria, they would need to meet a high standard of epistemic certainty given the inductive risks involved. Consciousness would fail, especially in the hard cases involving DoCs. In chapter 8, I turn to the disability critique of treatment withdrawals from DoC patients and consider the influence of ableism and bias on treatment and nontreatment decisions. The disability critique is important and warrants attention because it is informed by the way disabled persons are treated (and mistreated) in healthcare contexts. This chapter tugs further at threads found in previous chapters, including considerations of epistemic injustice, epistemic and moral duties, and the need for an all-things-considered approach to treatment decisions for DoC patients. The final chapter briefly surveys the possibilities for extending the ethics of uncertainty to other domains and dilemmas, vexing moral problems involving other contested cases, including nonhuman animals, and the problem of pain.

Much happened while I was writing this book, both in the science of DoCs and in my own life. I moved from a position as a philosophy professor at Michigan Technological University to Upstate Medical University and the Center for Bioethics and Humanities. There, I teach medical and health professions students and work in the hospital as an ethics consultant. Among the cases I have consulted on were some involving patients with devastating brain injuries, DoCs, and brain death. My understanding of how medical staff approach these injuries, these injured patients, and their families has been informed by that experience. It is important to know how difficult—in every possible way—it is for surrogates (who are usually family members), who face daunting and difficult choices about what to do while also confronting fear, grief, loss, and dire uncertainty. During my first year at Upstate, the SARS-CoV-2 pandemic descended on the world, and hospitals everywhere closed their doors to visitors. That made matters immeasurably more difficult and complicated for families and surrogates who struggled to make decisions for loved ones they could not even see, touch, or speak to directly. What is always hard became even harder. Witnessing this also hardened my commitment to be a ferocious advocate both for patients and for their families and surrogates, and to use whatever small influence and large privilege I have to that end. That commitment informs everything in the pages to follow.

L. Syd M Johnson
February 2021

PART I
LAYING THE GROUNDWORK

1

Consciousness

Consciousness has as many theories as theorists.
—Alan Cowey in "Current Awareness: Spotlight on
Consciousness"

1.1 Questions about Consciousness

Consciousness isn't a thing you can poke a stick at. It's not a natural kind, like a bit of quartz, or quarks, or water. Like life, which can be attributed to many entities but is not a thing with reality apart from living entities, consciousness can be attributed to conscious entities without being some further thing or fact, some mysterious, mentalizing "force" that can exist without conscious entities. It is manifested in conscious states and creatures but isn't a thing in and of itself. One of the enduring puzzles about consciousness and conscious states is how they, as apparently mental, nonphysical states, can manifest in a physical entity like a brain. We can point to a physical bit of brain, to a neuron, or a structure like the thalamus, but we can't locate consciousness within that bit of brain or its neural cells.

Consciousness is notoriously difficult to define. We might mean several different things when we speak of consciousness. We might mean, when we say that my cat Mal is conscious, that he is *sentient*, a creature capable of sensing and responding to his world, of feeling pain and pleasure. When Jeremy Bentham spoke of the importance of sentience to moral considerability, he declared that "The question is not, Can they reason? nor, Can they talk? but, Can they suffer?"

4 THE ETHICS OF UNCERTAINTY

(Bentham 1789). But we might look at Mal, snoozing in a sunbeam, and say, "He's unconscious," because he is asleep. *Wakefulness*, or a capacity for wakefulness, is sometimes what is meant by consciousness, and we might think that this kind of consciousness admits of degrees—perhaps that drowsy, semi-aware state we're in as we're falling asleep or waking up is a level of consciousness apart from the fully alert, eyes-open state we're in after two shots of espresso. Perhaps when we're dreaming, we're in another state or level of consciousness.

We could also mean by consciousness *self-consciousness* or *self-awareness*. This seems a more demanding way of thinking about consciousness, one that requires that Mal not only be awake and aware, but also aware that he is aware. Self-awareness is a kind of meta-awareness that involves an explicit conceptual awareness of oneself, awareness that what one experiences is being experienced by oneself, and a capacity to think about it. It might require diachronic identity, a durable sense of self as distinct from other things or creatures. As John Locke described it, such a creature would be "a thinking intelligent Being, that has reason and reflection, and can consider it self as itself, the same thinking thing in different times and places" (Locke 1689). The existence of this kind of awareness seems especially likely in the case of very intelligent, social mammals like elephants, orcas, and nonhuman primates, for whom self-awareness would enhance capacities for social coordination and theory of mind. When Mal watches a spider crawling up the wall and plans how he might catch the spider, he could be aware that he is thinking about the spider and thinking about himself thinking about the spider. Perhaps he thinks, "If I think about this some more, I'll figure out how to catch that spider." Again, in an important sense, this is a mental capacity rather than something one consciously does on the regular. There are very many things a creature like you or me or Mal does that don't require this kind of meta-awareness, including, perhaps, planning the capture or removal of a spider. It is likely that self-awareness of this sort is beyond the capacities of some humans, such as infants (and, if so, an interesting question is how and when it develops). It is also possible it is a capacity that some nonhuman animals do not have.

A less demanding kind of self-consciousness or awareness might be possible, a rudimentary and implicit sense of being the subject of experiences, such as being the subject of an itch, of feeling itchy. When David Hume looked inside his mind to find the *self*, he claimed he could not find it. What he saw therein was a rapid succession of images, passions, sensations, perceptions. He declared that those perceptions and sensations—the bundle of successive images and feelings—were all that constituted a person, and that he himself "never can catch myself at any time without a perception, and never can observe any thing but the perception" (Hume 1739). Self-awareness in the demanding sense described above is at best an illusion for Hume, something one might stitch together from assorted perceptions and feelings and infer a continuing subject, a self that is the subject of those percepts. But perhaps the second, less demanding sense of self-awareness is possible for Hume—an awareness of those inner experiences, thoughts, and perceptions that can be examined and thought about, percepts one can sense are one's own without being able to locate oneself in them.

There is a subjective quality to conscious states, what Thomas Nagel called the *what it is like* aspect that defines a creature as conscious if there is *something it is like to be that creature*, some subjective way that the world appears or feels from that creature's point of view. Nagel's example is bats. There is something it is like to be a bat, to use echolocation to hunt and to navigate. Bat consciousness— the qualitative feel of what it's like to be a bat—is something that a human, experiencing the world from a subjective human point of view, cannot understand. Peter Godfrey-Smith thinks that subjectivity is both ubiquitous in living things and partly constitutive of selves. "Subjectivity involves feelings and seemings; agency is doing and initiating. All living things (or all living things composed of cells) exhibit something like subjectivity and agency, but these features take a different form in the animal case" (Godfrey-Smith 2020, 104).

There are numerous questions we could ask about consciousness. Some of those questions are descriptive, questions like *What is consciousness? What are its features? How can it be discovered or detected?* These are questions that are both ontological, seeking to understand and describe the nature of consciousness, and epistemological, seeking to understand what and how we can know about consciousness. There are additional ontological questions, such as explanatory questions about how consciousness exists, how it occurs or arises in conscious creatures, and whether it is something with independent reality apart from conscious creatures. There are also functional questions about consciousness, questions about what consciousness does: *Does it have adaptive functions that might explain, for example, how and why consciousness is such a widespread phenomenon across numerous taxa and species?* This is also an origins question: *When/how/why did consciousness occur?* Functional questions about the role or importance of consciousness also have an ethical dimension. As Bentham claimed, whether a creature is sentient is all that *matters morally*. Robert van Gulick (2018) noted that "We are inclined to regard an organism's moral status as at least partly determined by the nature and extent to which it is conscious." A very strong claim about the *value* of consciousness, one that appears widely shared, was expressed by Daniel Bor:

Consciousness is required for all meaningful experiences. Consequently, many ethical questions, including the withdrawal of life support in disorders of patients with [disorders of consciousness], are underpinned by that person's capacity for consciousness. Unlocking the nature of consciousness, therefore, is one of the most profound issues remaining in biology. (2016)

The ethical questions about consciousness include questions about what sorts of consciousness have or don't have value, and why.

The ontological and epistemological questions are interesting. They are also importantly separate from ethical questions concerning conscious entities, by which I mean that we could answer all the ontological and epistemological questions about consciousness and there would still be unanswered ethical questions. But suppose we defined consciousness and identified all the conscious or possibly conscious entities. Suppose further that we had very good methods for discerning when a creature had lost consciousness, and whether there was any possibility of its regaining consciousness. That would not answer any *ethical* questions about consciousness, which include *Does consciousness matter morally? Does moral status depend on consciousness?* Certainty about which entities are conscious matters if we think that consciousness matters morally, or if we think what we ought to do is informed by whether an entity is conscious. The belief that consciousness is in some sense constitutive of persons or that consciousness defines one's moral status is widespread and is hardly questioned. I think it should be questioned. Knowing that an entity is conscious answers ethical questions only if we have already answered prior questions about the moral significance of consciousness. And how well we can know that some entity is conscious should figure into our considerations about the significance of consciousness to ethical questions about how we ought to treat entities identified as conscious or unconscious.

Renewed interest in the scientific and philosophical study of consciousness emerged in the 1980s and 1990s. There has amassed since a vast literature, which I do not plan to canvas here. Neither is it my intention to offer a detailed map of the terrain—that work has been done capably elsewhere. Rather, to extend the map metaphor, I aim only to present a rough sketch of the lay of the land, with particular attention to the features that are relevant to the present project.

1.2 A Side Note about Other Minds

The problem of other minds is an epistemological problem famously associated with René Descartes, who, in the course of arriving at a radical methodological skepticism about sensory perception in the *Meditations*, concluded that the only thing he could know was that he himself was thinking. He could not know that there were other things that exist, and lacking direct access to other minds, he could not know that there were other minds. Descartes also famously (or infamously) concluded that nonhuman animals do not have souls and are not conscious but are mere automatons (*bête machine*). When they writhed and screamed as he cut them open, their actions could not be attributed to the existence of an incorporeal, rational soul, or self-consciousness.[1] Of course, Descartes fell into solipsism—he had no reason to attribute the behaviors of other humans—humans other than himself—as signs of a rational soul or consciousness either. Centuries on, it is obvious that other beings exhibit many of the behaviors that, in humans, we take to be signs of consciousness. Dogs clearly use their sensitive olfactory sense to navigate the world, and their sensitive hearing to detect the sound of a can being opened at the other end of the house. They act purposefully, respond to their environments, communicate their needs and desires, demonstrate emotions and emotional awareness, and even appear to be moral agents with a sense of justice. The debate over teleost fish pain is over (although there are still some skeptical holdouts). Teleost fish feel pain. They also cooperate, interact, solve problems, and respond to their environments. Yet there remains skepticism about animal consciousness, despite considerable evidence that very many animals are conscious. Perhaps such

---

[1] Whether Descartes positively asserted that animals could not feel pain is a matter of debate. His conclusions about their lack of soul or consciousness might also have been his skepticism at work—he never found a rational argument to prove otherwise (see, for example, Harrison 1992). The ethical implications of such an epistemological stance are staggering.

skepticism is less informed by empirical evidence of animal consciousness, which is at least as strong as evidence for general human consciousness, than by religious and cultural beliefs, and mundane practicalities like the use of animals for food and scientific research.

1.3 The Lay of the Land: An Incomplete Sketch of Theories of Consciousness

> The fundamental question at the heart of the mind–body problem is, *what is the relation between the conscious mind and the electro-chemical interactions in the body that give rise to it?* How do the salty taste and crunchy texture of potato chips, the unmistakable smell of dogs after they have been in the rain, or the feeling of hanging on tiny fingerholds on a cliff a couple of meters above the last secure foothold, emerge from networks of neurons? (Koch 2004, 1)

Descartes' theory of consciousness or mind was *substance dualism*—he thought that the mind or soul was an immaterial substance, while the body was a physical substance. How the immaterial and material interacted—how the mind interacts with the body—was a question he could not satisfactorily answer. Substance dualism is largely out of favor at present. *Property dualism*, of which there are several flavors, posits the existence of conscious properties that are not identical with, nor reducible to, physical properties (e.g., brain states or processes), but are instantiated by the same things (brains, neurons) that instantiate those physical properties. One variety of property dualism is emergent property dualism, which treats consciousness or conscious states as arising from complex physical systems or organizations. The resulting *mental* properties are, as it were, greater than the sum of the physical parts from which they emerge, and they are distinctly different from the physical. Property dualism runs afoul of the Hard Problem of Consciousness, so named by David Chalmers. The Hard Problem is the problem of explaining why any physical state is *conscious* rather than nonconscious, how it is, as T. H. Huxley said, "that anything so remarkable as a state of consciousness comes about as a result of irritating nervous tissue" (Huxley 1890). It is the problem of explaining why there is "something it is like" for a subject of conscious experience.

The qualitative nature of consciousness—how it feels to be conscious—is not merely another way of categorizing states of the brain or of behavior. Levine calls this the "explanatory gap" between the physical brain and subjective experience, which points to one of the most vexing and wide-ranging puzzles about consciousness.[2]

Panpsychism is a type of property dualism that regards all constituents of reality as having some psychic properties distinct from their physical properties. Some neuroscientists endorse a form of panpsychism, such as Giulio Tononi's integrated information theory (IIT) of consciousness. According to IIT, consciousness is identical with integrated information within a network system and admits of degrees. IIT allows that both simple systems (diodes) and complex systems (humans, robots, computers) can be conscious, hence the panpsychism. IIT is compatible with the observation that the injured brains of humans with disorders of consciousness (DoCs) can exhibit intact activity in some regions of the brain that are disconnected and therefore not integrated. We might wonder if there is a global state of consciousness in such a disconnected brain, or if there are conscious contents that permit a kind of local level of consciousness, an assortment of unbundled percepts, feelings, and emotions.

---

[2] The explanatory gap can be cashed out in different ways. In its weakest form, it simply states that there is a practical limit to our explanatory capabilities given current understanding, but in principle the gap can be closed. A stronger form asserts that it is in principle impossible to bridge the gap given the limits of human cognitive capacities, or that it is in principle impossible for any cognitive agents to bridge the gap.

Physicalists/materialists about consciousness claim that consciousness can be explained entirely in terms of certain physical properties or states of the brain (e.g., thalamocortical connections or activity in the prefrontal parietal network [PPN]). Here again, the question of how it is that conscious experiences have a qualitative feel (or qualia) emerges. What explains the "what-it's-likeness" of conscious experience if consciousness amounts to the firing of neurons, or activations of the PPN? Where is the sweet scent of a rose or the sour taste of a lemon to be found in the firing of neurons? Some physicalists endorse type–type identity and deny that there is an explanatory gap or anything further to explain. Conscious qualitative properties and neural properties are simply identical, and there is no need to explain how the latter causes the former. There is no cause and effect. Everything is identical with itself, and so, too, are conscious qualitative properties and neural properties—there is no need to explain such an identity relation.

One variety of physicalist theory is neural theories, which seek to identify the neural (or neuronal) correlates of consciousness (NCCs). Francis Crick and Christof Koch defined a neuronal correlate of consciousness as a "minimal set of neuronal events and mechanisms jointly sufficient for a specific conscious percept" (Koch 2004, 16). Consciousness might refer to overall states of background consciousness (e.g., being awake, dreaming) or more fine-grained content-consciousness. NCCs are *sufficient* but not necessary for specific conscious states because there might be multiple NCCs of any given conscious state (e.g., a headache, a craving for coffee; Chalmers 2000). Koch argued that there must be explicit correspondence between a mental event and its neuronal correlates, such that a change in one must be associated with a change in the other. Importantly, NCCs are *correlated* with consciousness but need not be dedicated to, or constitutive of, consciousness. A given NCC may not be responsible for generating consciousness, but some NCCs might be essential for consciousness. Disruption or loss of those properties or processes—such as damage to consciousness-essential structures in the brain—might explain DoCs. Lesion studies of disordered brains thus provide several clues to NCCs. In DoCs, the lack of white matter integrity in the thalamus has been correlated with the vegetative state/unresponsive wakefulness syndrome (VS/UWS; Fernández-Espejo et al. 2011). Metabolic dysfunction and functional disconnectivity in the frontoparietal network are correlated with the loss of awareness in the VS/UWS (Laureys 2005). Studies of lesions to the PPN also suggest the PPN's essential role in conscious awareness (Bor 2016). The global neuronal workspace (GNW) theory posits that domain-specific local processing is the source of conscious *contents*, but conscious access/awareness occurs only when they are integrated into a global workspace involving the PPN. GNW, IIT, and a number of other hypotheses are consistent with experimental findings that indicate that consciousness requires sustained, complex, differentiated, and brain-scale communication (Naccache 2017).

I find it plausible that consciousness is a system-level feature of the brain, and a multiply realizable property of physical organisms. Conscious and mental properties *emerge* through the aggregate functions of a sufficiently complex and connected system like a brain. That does not mean that the system must be a brain, although all the creatures known to be conscious in the way that humans are conscious have a brain or central nervous system. I suspect that to view consciousness as a property of brains alone is too limited—consciousness in some creatures, like cephalopods, may well be as or more embodied than embrained. But to say (as I think is plausible) that consciousness and conscious states are not identical with physical states, and are not further facts about the physical world, but emerge out of interactions within sufficiently complex physical organisms, does not actually solve the Hard Problem nor close the explanatory gap. It is in no way an explanation of what consciousness is, or how it actually emerges in terrestrial (or, presumably, extraterrestrial) organisms. It leaves unanswered the ontological questions, but answering those questions is not my project.

Nonetheless, the ontological questions will end up mattering as we proceed, in part because they contribute to uncertainty about consciousness, and the uncertainty of consciousness across several domains is a key theme, and a key problem, that this book addresses. Part of that uncertainty results from not knowing exactly what it is we mean by consciousness in the neurological or neuroscientific sense, and in the context of personhood and moral status.

> The concept of consciousness is a hybrid or better, a mongrel concept: the word 'consciousness' connotes a number of different concepts and denotes a number of different phenomena. We reason about "consciousness" using some premises that apply to one of the phenomena that fall under "consciousness," other premises that apply to other "consciousnesses" and we end up with trouble. (Block 2002)

Ned Block differentiated between phenomenal and access consciousness (and these make a return appearance later, in the chapter on moral status). Phenomenal consciousness, or P-consciousness, is described above as experience that has a what-it's-like aspect, to it. That is, P-consciousness *is experience*, and what makes it phenomenally conscious is that there's something it's like to be in a state of P-consciousness. That's a circular definition, which Block has readily admitted (Block 2002). Access, or A-consciousness, has representational contents like beliefs, thoughts, and desires that are available for "use in reasoning and for direct 'rational' control of action (including reporting)" (Block 1995). The contents of P-consciousness (e.g., feeling itchy) can also be A-conscious (e.g., motivating scratching).

1.4 Consciousness, Disordered

If we set aside the problem of other minds, it is often apparent to us when a human is conscious. They respond to their environment—to voices, sights, sounds, the mosquito that has landed on their arm, and other sensations. They behave purposefully. They swat away the mosquito. They move to turn up the radio when their favorite song is playing. They have ideas about what songs they like. They sing along. They can also do things like think, speak, solve puzzles, read books, and follow the plot—the plot of their life, or the plot of a movie. They cry out in pain, cry with happiness, feel sad, angry, happy. The reader will have noted here that all the evidence for consciousness cited thus far is behavioral. Conscious humans behave as if there is something going on inside, something unseen. They're not automatons, clockwork toys, or robots programmed to act like humans. The unseen inside—consciousness—remains obscure and ambiguous. More on that in a minute.

The astute reader will also have noticed that there are humans who cannot (or cannot yet, or cannot anymore) perform some of the behaviors that signal consciousness. Infants can cry out in pain, but they don't behave purposefully, solve puzzles, speak, or follow plots. Someone with advanced dementia might no longer be able to follow the plot of their lives or a movie, or read a book. One need not exhibit all of these behaviors for us to be reasonably certain that one is conscious. Reasonably certain because what is going on inside is what we think of as "consciousness," but what is going on outside is what serves as our evidence. Consciousness is not like cardiac activity. We can hear the heart beating. We can see the heart beating if we cut your chest open, or use ultrasound. We can also see indirect evidence of the heart beating, in the blood coursing through the body, the pulse, the activity of an electrocardiogram. Not so consciousness. Although consciousness is usually thought to be a function of the brain, and we can "see" brain activity through active imaging (e.g., on an electroencephalogram, or with functional magnetic resonance imaging), and can locate that activity, that doesn't get us to consciousness. Brain activity is, at best, a proxy for consciousness.

In the context of DoCs, the *what* of consciousness is clinically described in operational terms of *wakefulness* (or arousal, vigilance) and *awareness*. Wakefulness refers to brain activity and states, or the presence of sleep/wake cycles. Awareness refers to the contents of consciousness—self-awareness and awareness of the external world. Of the two, awareness is the more demanding, and the two types of awareness, of the self and of the external world, are distinct. Many creatures are thought to be sentient and aware of the external world. They are able to sense and to respond to things in their environments. As noted above, self-awareness can be more or less demanding, depending on the extent to which it requires meta-awareness. Within the definitions of DoCs, wakefulness is compatible with impaired consciousness—those in a coma do not awaken, while those in the VS/UWS and the minimally conscious state (MCS) do. Thus, while different DoCs are defined and differentiated in part by the presence of states of wakefulness, wakefulness is less relevant to defining consciousness itself. Conscious creatures do, after all, sleep and lose consciousness from time to time, so wakefulness is more usefully thought of as a *capacity* for wakefulness or arousal, and one that is shared by typically and nontypically functioning brains and across the brains of many species.

In coma, there is neither wakefulness nor awareness. In the VS/UWS, there is eyes-open wakefulness without self or external awareness. VS/UWS patients are unresponsive to stimuli, except for reflexive responses. From the outside, they look and behave as if they are unaware. Patients in the MCS are responsive, with more than reflexive responses to external stimuli. From the outside, they can look and behave as if they are aware, although this behavior is less consistent than it is in typically functioning individuals. What it means to be "minimally conscious" is a bit of a puzzle—it implies that consciousness is not all or nothing, that there can be levels or degrees of consciousness, perhaps like the difference between being fully awake and alert and the twilight drowsiness of falling asleep. Because there remains uncertainty about consciousness, and whether particular individuals are conscious, there is a potential mismatch between the names that have been given to DoCs and the syndromes themselves. This much is true: individual patients are behaviorally responsive or unresponsive (or their brains are responsive or unresponsive—more on that later), and their behavioral responsiveness indicates which diagnostic category they are assigned to, which may or may not accurately reflect what's going on inside.

If, as Block has argued, consciousness is not a unitary concept but a "mongrel" denoting different concepts or varieties, if you will, of consciousness, that would be important in the context of DoCs. In the next chapter, I consider whether there is indeed this kind of confusion about consciousnesses, such that there is a mismatch between clinical diagnostic tools and the thing—global consciousness—they purport to detect.

1.5 A Funny Thing about Conscious Creatures

Most of us have had the experience of leaping into action to prevent some large or small mishap—catching a glass just before it hits the floor, grabbing a child before they fall into a pool, slamming on the brakes when a squirrel suddenly dodges into the road. We can do those things without thinking or planning. If we had to plan or think first, we'd be too slow to react.

A whole whack of things that humans do they do without conscious awareness. There has been abundant research on this, both in persons with brain anomalies (like blindsight[3]) and in typically

___

[3] Blindsight is the ability of persons with visual field defects caused by damage to the primary visual cortex to detect, localize, and even discriminate visual stimuli despite

functioning humans. It seems a rather useful feature of our lives and our brains. If we had to consciously attend to every detail of every purposeful action, we would need either radically faster, higher bandwidth brains, or we would have to slow way down. Imagine having to consciously attend to every minute movement while driving. We tap the brakes just so, turn the wheel just so, step a little harder on the accelerator without having to be consciously aware of needing to do those things, or of doing them. And once we learn a route, we don't have to consciously look for landmarks or signs as we do when we're driving somewhere for the first time. This gives us more flexibility, the ability to improvise, the ability to turn our attention to the song on the radio or the conversation we're having. For a beginning driver, it is all much harder because it requires more will, more thought, more conscious cognition.

Experiments have revealed a number of other things humans can do without explicit conscious awareness, including "correlate information, associate meanings, reason in a very fast way, develop complex computations, perform sophisticated mathematical operations, selectively focus on information, [and] develop complex inferences" (Farisco and Evers 2017). They can also have unconscious emotions—not only emotional responses that are unconsciously triggered, but also unconscious emotional reactions intense enough to alter their behavior, in the absence of conscious feelings (Winkielman and Berridge 2004). An astonishing example of unconscious action is sleepwalking. Somnambulists perform complex actions—walking, eating, driving cars, and reportedly even committing homicides—while asleep and wholly unaware.[4] Some absence seizures also appear to involve consciousness

being phenomenally unaware of them (Cowey 2010). Blindsight has also been experimentally verified in monkeys (Cowey and Stoerig 1995).

[4] Somnambulism occurs during the deepest stages of NREM, or non-rapid eye movement sleep. During episodes, the sleepwalking individual appears awake but is unresponsive, and sensory perceptions are virtually switched off, so sleepwalkers do not fully perceive sight, smell, sound, or even pain, but they can nonetheless perform sometimes quite complex actions, as in this case:

without awareness (Blumenfeld 2005). Persons undergoing absence seizures can sometimes engage in perceptual-driven motor responses (e.g., finger-tapping, turning the head to look at someone), but have limited capacities for reasoning and memory consolidation.

Some conclude from the frequency of action without awareness in humans that animals are not conscious because, although they can perform complex tasks and actions (watch the ball, chase the ball, find the ball, return the ball), those tasks can be performed without conscious awareness. I think this is the wrong conclusion to draw. The fact that we *can* perform even complex actions and tasks below the threshold of conscious awareness (or while asleep) does not mean that creatures without consciousness can perform the same feats. Consciousness "under the hood" may be necessary for nonrandom, nonreflexive, complex actions. I may be able to successfully drive a familiar route home without being aware of every movement and adjustment I have to perform, but it's not plausible that I could do it unless I were a conscious creature who could become aware of, and consciously control, my actions.

The dissociation between awareness and nonreflexive action may have interesting implications for DoCs, a point I return to in the next chapter.

> During the night of May 23, 1987, Kenneth Parks rose from his bed and wandered out of his house and into his car, driving 14 miles to the home of his mother- and father-in-law in the neighboring town. Upon arriving at their home, he took a tire iron from the car and entered the house. He then beat his mother-in-law to death and choked his father-in-law. Now a blood-spattered mess covered in cuts and bruises, he drove to a nearby police station. In a confused manner, he told the police that he "thought" he killed someone. Though still confused, he identified his in-laws, murmuring that it was "all his fault." Eventually, Parks was tried for one charge of murder and one charge of attempted murder. His defense claimed that, during the entire episode, he was sleepwalking. (Popat and Winslade 2015, 204)

Parks was also found to have highly irregular EEG results and no motive for killing his in-laws, and he was acquitted of murder and attempted murder.

2

Unconsciousness

If names be not correct, language is not in accordance with the truth of things.

—*The Analects Attributed to Confucius,*
551–479 BCE by Lao-Tse

2.1 The Disorders of Consciousness

The modern era of disorders of consciousness (DoCs) began with the advent of intensive care measures that kept apneic, comatose patients alive, especially the small, tracheal positive-pressure ventilators developed in the 1950s. Prior to that, there are references to conditions resembling these disorders dating back centuries, including in the works of Hippocrates and Galen, although the inability to keep alive those who were unable to breathe or take nourishment would have made such patients exceedingly rare, and their lives exceedingly short. DoCs can result from acquired brain injuries or from progressive neurodegenerative disorders. Because these disorders have a variety of causes, including localized injuries to different areas of the brain, and different etiologies, including traumatic, ischemic, and hypoxic/anoxic brain injuries, as well as neurodegenerative conditions like Tay-Sachs and Alzheimer's dementia, no two patients are exactly alike. The current diagnostic categories were developed over several decades as medical experience with these disorders accumulated and it became clear that patients existed with a spectrum of impairments.

2.1.1 Behavioral Distinctions

> Consciousness is a state that is elusive and not necessarily
> directly measurable. In the clinical context, assessing the
> presence of consciousness in a patient is based on prag-
> matic principles in which a patient can demonstrate vol-
> untary/purposeful behaviors that can be taken to imply a
> state of (at least minimal) consciousness. (Provencio et al.
> 2020)

DoCs are diagnosed and classified behaviorally, in terms of the type
and quality of responsiveness demonstrated by patients. Owing to
the distinctive heterogeneity of brain injuries, patients with quite
different underlying pathologies can satisfy *behavioral* criteria for
the same DoC. The differences in pathology can include etiology
and location/severity of lesions, as well as variable preservation of
different mental states (Johnson and Lazaridis 2018). But specific
sensory, motoric, and cognitive impairments can confound behavioral diagnosis. Thus, DoCs as *diagnostic* classifications do not
pick out natural kinds with respect to consciousness or conscious
content (Klein 2015). In recent years, there have been calls to further refine and reform the taxonomy of DoCs, in part because of
uncertainties caused by the poor fit between the behavioral criteria
used to diagnose DoCs and the phenomena—consciousness and
mentality—purportedly being diagnosed (Bayne, Hohwy, and
Owen 2017; Provencio et al. 2020).

Outward behaviors are coarse-grained proxies for what lies
within—but they are proxies with some diagnostic utility. It's reasonable to ask, however, if we should continue to classify or *define*
disorders using strictly behavioral criteria knowing how frequently
they miss the mark, and knowing how serious and consequential
misdiagnosis can be. As Tim Bayne et al. have argued, "The exclusive reliance on behavior would be justified if consciousness was a
behavioral phenomenon, but it is not" (2017, 867).

2.1.2   Coma

Coma is a state of unconsciousness in which a patient lacks any awareness of self or the external world. The comatose individual shows no signs of wakefulness or eye opening, no purposeful behaviors, no language or response to commands, and no vocalizations. The individual in a coma also typically has impaired brainstem reflexes and cannot breathe without the aid of a ventilator. A variety of outcomes are possible, including recovery of consciousness, progression to another DoC, or death.

2.1.3   The Vegetative State/Unresponsive Wakefulness Syndrome

In 1972, Bryan Jennett and Fred Plum coined the term *persistent vegetative state* (PVS) to describe patients who awaken from coma into a state of chronic unresponsiveness (Jennett and Plum 1972). The vegetative state (VS) was previously referred to by several names, including *apallic syndrome, akinetic mutism,* and *coma vigile.* More recently, there have been calls to change the name of this disorder to unresponsive wakefulness syndrome (UWS).[1] The patient in the VS/UWS exhibits arousal or wakefulness and has sleep/wake cycles and periods of eye opening. That is, they have one of the components of consciousness—wakefulness or arousal—but show no signs of the other component, *awareness.* They have no nonreflexive responses to stimuli and show no behavioral evidence

---

[1] UWS has had more uptake in Europe than in North America and elsewhere. There are important definitional differences between UWS and VS, the most significant being that UWS is agnostic concerning whether an individual is conscious or unconscious, while VS is a diagnosis of unconsciousness. Indeed, one motive for shifting to UWS is that it describes the behavioral symptoms—the patient is unresponsive—without inferring unconsciousness. That VS and UWS are used together acknowledges that they refer to the same syndrome, although they are in tension concerning the absence of consciousness.

of conscious awareness of the self or the external world. They can vocalize, but there is no apparent language comprehension or response to commands, and no purposeful behavior. Typically, brainstem reflexes are preserved, and the VS/UWS patient is able to breathe on their own (Heine, Laureys, and Schnakers 2016), although they are dependent on tube feeding.

Twenty-two years after the PVS was named and defined, temporal criteria were established to distinguish the *persistent* vegetative state from the *permanent* vegetative state (Multi-Society Task Force 1994). By then, it was understood that some patients do recover from the VS, and some do not. At the time, the VS was considered permanent and irreversible 3 months after an anoxic/hypoxic brain injury, and 12 months after a traumatic brain injury.[2] The difference is due to the improved chances of recovery for those with localized traumatic brain injuries as compared to patients with the widespread brain injury typical after an anoxic or hypoxic event. Once the threshold for permanence was crossed, the chance of recovering consciousness was thought to be vanishingly small, nearing impossibility.

Unfortunately, the *persistent* and the *permanent* VS have the same initials, which continues to cause confusion among the public and popular press. The temporally, diagnostically, prognostically, and ethically distinct states are frequently conflated in the bioethics literature as well. This is not merely a failure to keep current on esoteric terminology. The persistent VS is, by definition, a temporary, time-limited condition in which recovery remains possible. To fail to recognize this when discussing, for example, the moral status or personhood of these patients or the withdrawal of life-sustaining treatment is to ignore ethically salient facts.

---

[2] In the United Kingdom, the VS is considered permanent 6 months after an anoxic/hypoxic injury.

Recent studies have cast doubt on the temporal boundaries for permanence and recovery in the VS/UWS. Studies that followed patients longitudinally found that recovery and improvement can continue for several years post-injury. For that reason, a terminological change to *chronic* VS/UWS has been recommended (Giacino et al. 2018) to replace *permanent* VS/UWS, in recognition of the continued potential for recovery of consciousness, as well as the stability and chronicity of the disorder.

Unresponsive wakefulness syndrome was proposed as a new name for the VS in 2010 by the European Task Force on Disorders of Consciousness (Laureys et al. 2010). The change was proposed for several reasons: (1) to reduce the stigma associated with the term *vegetative*, which has taken on a pejorative, less-than-human connotation; (2) to acknowledge the high rate of misdiagnosis of the VS, as well as recent evidence that some unresponsive patients are conscious (UWS describes the patient as unresponsive, but does not imply unconsciousness); (3) to adopt a more clinically descriptive but metaphysically and ethically neutral term (Laureys et al. 2010). I agree that UWS is a more appropriate term. However, we are currently in a transitional time in which the understanding of DoCs and their taxonomy remains in flux, and others have proposed even further refinements of the DoC taxonomy (Naccache 2017; Bayne, Hohwy, and Owen 2017), which may result in further terminological refinements being proposed or adopted in the future. Throughout this book, I use VS/UWS preferentially. I think it is more appropriate, given the potential for misdiagnosis of unconsciousness and the behavioral nature of the diagnostic criteria, to use the term *unresponsive*. But I also use VS alone at times when referring to discussions that predate recent discoveries and developments. Because UWS is agnostic regarding the presence or absence of consciousness, it really is not equivalent to VS, which is a diagnosis of unconsciousness. It would confuse the issue to retroactively change references to the PVS wherein it is assumed that it is a state of unconsciousness.

2.1.4 The Minimally Conscious State

In 2002, 30 years after the VS was named and defined, the minimally conscious state (MCS) was defined to describe patients who emerged from the VS into a condition of partial or diminished awareness (Giacino et al. 2002). Patients in the MCS exhibit inconsistent and minimal but definite and reproducible behavioral evidence of awareness. The MCS is subcategorized into the MCS- and the MCS+ to mark two behaviorally different levels of disability. Patients in the MCS- exhibit low levels of behavioral responsiveness, such as visual fixation or visual pursuit (that is, being able to look at or follow an object with their eyes), localization to pain (trying to remove a painful stimulus), or appropriate responses to emotional stimuli. MCS+ patients exhibit higher-level responses, including command following, object recognition, intelligible verbalizations, or intentional communication, such as yes/no gesturing, and appropriate emotional responses to environmental stimuli (Bruno et al. 2011).[3] Emergence from the MCS (EMCS) is marked by the return of functional and reliable (verbal or gestural) communication and of the functional use of objects (Monti 2015).

Neuroimaging studies have yielded empirical evidence of pain perception and the potential for suffering, as well as emotional response, in the MCS (Schnakers et al. 2010, 2012; Bekinschtein et al. 2004). Caroline Schnakers et al. have developed a Nociception Coma Scale to assess pain behaviors in DoCs. The scale involves observation of motor, verbal, and visual responses and facial expressions in response to painful stimuli (Schnakers et al. 2012). It appears likely that MCS patients, but not VS/UWS patients, can experience pain. Using positron emission tomography (PET),

---

[3] The MCS was only added to the International Classification of Diseases (ICD-11) in September 2020, some two decades after it was formally defined. The lack of a standardized diagnostic code for MCS has hindered epidemiological, morbidity, and mortality data collection and has complicated medical reimbursement for this disorder.

Melanie Boly et al. studied brain activation induced by noxious stimulation of the median nerve:

> In patients in MCS and in controls, noxious stimulation activated the thalamus, S1, and the secondary somatosensory or insular, frontoparietal, and anterior cingulate cortices (known as the pain matrix). No area was less activated in the patients in MCS than in the controls. All areas of the cortical pain matrix showed greater activation in patients in MCS than in those in PVS. (2008, 1013)

Functional neuroimaging has also demonstrated language network activation in MCS patients (Giacino et al. 2020). This evidence reinforces the need to treat pain or distress, or perhaps to provide positive and enjoyable stimuli, to MCS patients. The presence of sentience and perhaps psychological/emotional states in the MCS adds complexity to ethical deliberations concerning these patients and has vexed legal deliberations as well.

With relatively minimal care, including tube feeding and basic nursing care, chronic VS/UWS and MCS patients can live for decades. Once discharged from hospital care, these patients can live in the community—either in the family home or in a long-term nursing facility. Recent studies show that about 20 percent of patients with prolonged DoCs will regain the capacities for independent living within 2 to 5 years of injury (Nakase-Richardson et al. 2012; Katz et al. 2009).

2.1.5 Cognitive Motor Dissociation

A notable development in DoCs involves the discovery, in the early 2000s, that some patients who appear on standard behavioral assessment to be unconscious are "covertly aware." They are able to respond to questions and commands through willful, self-directed control of their brain activity detectable only through neuroimaging (Cruse et al. 2011; Monti et al. 2010; Owen et al. 2006). This syndrome has been called *functional locked-in syndrome* (fLIS)[4] or cognitive motor dissociation (CMD; Schiff 2015), to designate individuals with extreme motor dysfunction and identifiable higher cognitive functions that are measurable only with functional neuroimaging. Monti et al. argued that functional neuroimaging can reveal "brain behaviors" that are otherwise covert and inaccessible, and that such brain activity is an objective and reliable indicator of consciousness (Monti et al. 2010).

CMD spans DoC categories and can include VS/UWS and MCS patients. It is less a diagnosis, in the traditional sense that means identifying a disease, condition, or injury from its signs and symptoms, and more a distinction based on *how* the diagnosis is made. This is not typical when defining disorders. We can diagnose a broken bone by clinical examination or by using an X-ray, but the diagnosis and treatment remain the same. It wouldn't make sense to differentiate between bone fractures based on how they are diagnosed. Bayne et al. argued that the CMD is problematic as a DoC category because it implies that "the distinction between patients whose conscious experiences are manifest in their overt behavior and patients whose conscious experiences are not overtly manifest is a fundamental one" (Bayne, Hohwy, and Owen 2017, 871). What is important, they argued, is not *how* patients manifest behavioral evidence of consciousness, but *whether they are conscious*.

The existence of CMD is, however, further confirmation of the shortcomings of behavioral diagnosis, and the mismatch between what is sought and what is actually caught by diagnosis. The

[4] fLIS is not to be confused with classic locked-in syndrome (LIS), which is not a DoC. Locked-in individuals experience total or near-total paralysis, typically from a brainstem lesion, but with no loss or impairment of consciousness. Some LIS patients retain the ability to blink their eyes and are able to communicate using assistive communication devices. LIS patients are sometimes misdiagnosed as being in the VS/UWS because they are unable to perform the behaviors that indicate they are conscious.

former is the confirmation of consciousness or unconsciousness, but behavioral diagnosis involves too much noise—the absence of selected behaviors can indicate an absence of consciousness, but it can also indicate specific sensory, motor, and cognitive deficits that tell us nothing about the overall awareness of the patient. The problem with behavioral diagnosis is that there is no mechanism for finding the meaningful signal in the noise. The use of neuroimaging has made it possible to detect a signal in a subset of patients, but it remains vulnerable to some of the same noise—deficits that impair brain responsiveness. The discovery of CMD patients has added to concerns about the problem of misdiagnosis of the VS/UWS. They are a cohort of patients highly vulnerable to behavior-based misdiagnosis, whose consciousness can only be detected through technological means that are expensive, and currently considered experimental, and therefore not widely accessible to patients outside of research studies.

2.1.6 Behavior Without Awareness

In chapter 1, I discuss the many things conscious creatures can do without conscious awareness, including performing complex, nonreflexive, environmentally interactive actions. As I said there, many of those actions are only possible for the kinds of creatures that *can* be conscious, even if some (perhaps a lot) of what they do is below the threshold of awareness. The dissociation between awareness and nonreflexive action suggests an interesting possibility for DoCs, and especially the VS/UWS. The fact that someone *does not* perform certain tasks or behaviors (e.g., tracking movement with one's eyes, localizing to pain, performing a mental task on command) in response to external stimuli may be just another way that awareness and action dissociate. In typically functioning humans, much of what goes on below the surface does not manifest in purposeful behaviors, but much purposeful behavior is also directed by brain activity not only below the surface, but below the level of subjective awareness. If awareness and complex, nonreflexive behaviors can dissociate in the one case—the case of conscious humans acting without awareness—that gives us one more reason to doubt that nonreflexive behaviors are informative concerning the absence of consciousness or awareness.[5]

2.2 From Epistemic Certainty to Uncertainty

It is difficult to overstate the ethical significance of the existence of the MCS and CMD. First, because some patients progress from the VS/UWS to the MCS or CMD, the very existence of these DoCs is proof that the VS is not always permanent, and not so certainly hopeless as once thought. Second, both MCS and CMD are further evidence of a significant problem of misdiagnosis—one that has resisted improvement for decades. The rate of misdiagnosis in DoCs is estimated to be between 39 and 43 percent (Schnakers et al. 2009; van Erp et al. 2015). This would be unacceptably high in any area of medicine, but it is of special concern with DoCs, where there is a false negative error in which patients are diagnosed as unconscious (because evidence of consciousness is not found) when they are in fact conscious. The error occurs because the MCS can be exceedingly difficult to distinguish from the VS/UWS based on behavior alone. CMD patients, similarly, exhibit no purposeful overt behaviors that would distinguish them from VS/UWS or MCS

---

[5] Michele Farisco and Kathinka Evers argued that "the unconscious is ethically relevant" and may require reevaluation of diagnostic strategies to assess for "residual unconscious activities" (Farisco and Evers 2017). In particular, they raised concerns about the potential for unconscious positive and negative emotions, and the possibility of unconscious processing of information and stimuli. Farisco and Evers are convinced that unconscious emotions of which one is phenomenally unaware affect well-being. Given the damaging effects of chronic stress (including unaware stress) on health and well-being, there are reasons to be concerned about patients living in care environments in which aversive and negative emotional experiences (e.g., loneliness, pain, boredom) might be common.

patients. But diagnostic and prognostic error can prompt limitations or withdrawals of treatment for patients, in the belief that further care will be of no benefit. It can also result in patients being effectively warehoused in nursing homes, where, on the belief that they are unconscious, they receive care that keeps them alive but doesn't enhance their potential for improvement. Should they experience a "covert" recovery, they may not have opportunities for a new diagnosis. The diagnosis of unconsciousness or minimal consciousness can thus result in a self-fulfilling or self-reinforcing prophecy of hopelessness.

DoCs are somewhat paradoxical. As knowledge of these disorders has developed since the 1970s, and the diagnostic categories have expanded, one might expect that certainty about DoCs would correspondingly increase. It has instead gone the other way, ushering in a new age of uncertainty.

2.3 The Vegetative State: The Fateful Label

In naming the vegetative state, Jennett and Plum sought to describe a syndrome that could be diagnosed behaviorally at the bedside, and that would not imply any particular etiology or lesion. They fatefully adopted the term *vegetative* from archaic usage in the *Oxford English Dictionary* to describe "an organic body capable of growth and development but devoid of sensation and thought (1764)," and *vegetate*, meaning "to live a merely physical life, devoid of intellectual activity or social intercourse (1740)" (Jennett and Plum 1972). The term *vegetative* had been used informally for a century to describe patients in a coma-like state, but its etymological roots date back to at least Aristotle, who in *De Anima* (Aristotle 1941, Book II, 413a23) described the soul as a nested, hierarchical set of capacities found in living things. According to Aristotle, the nutritive (or vegetative) soul is present in all living things (plants, animals, and humans). Animals have nutritive and sensitive souls and are capable of sensation. The rational soul, the intellectual soul, is found only in humans, and enables distinctly human capacities (in addition to the capacities of the nutritive and sensitive soul). While modern English speakers associate the term *vegetative* with vegetables or plants, its roots, so to speak, point to the distinction between being alive and being conscious and capable of thought. It distinguishes, in other words, between mere biological life and life that is distinctly human and rational (and, hence, specially valuable). And so Jennett and Plum intended for the term to indicate to doctors a condition in which autonomic (vegetative) functions continue while "the cerebral cortex is not functioning," and they sought terminology that laypersons could understand. Unfortunately, the term quickly took on a more pejorative connotation, as patients were (and continue to be) referred to as "vegetables," implying that they were less than human, perhaps even less than alive.

2.3.1   A Fate Worse Than Death? The Vegetative State and the Right to Die

Essentially, she's a cadaver with a heartbeat.[6]
There's a case there and somebody's taken the motherboard out.[7]

A mere 3 years after the Jennett and Plum paper was published, the Karen Ann Quinlan case emerged as a pivotal legal battle involving the right to die for PVS patients. Quinlan was a college student who fell into a coma and then a VS (at the time, known only as the *persistent* VS) after consuming an unlucky combination of drugs and alcohol at a party. After she had been in the persistent VS for

---

[6] A son, describing his mother, diagnosed in a persistent VS (from my case notes for a hospital ethics consult).
[7] A brother, describing his sibling, quoted in Holland, Kitzinger, and Kitzinger (2014).

a few months, her parents sought to have her ventilator removed, believing it would result in her death.[8] Quinlan's doctors refused. Quinlan's parents fought a nationally publicized legal battle in the state of New Jersey and eventually prevailed. Dr. Fred Plum, the court-appointed neurologist, testified in the case. In upholding the right of Quinlan's parents to withdraw life support, the New Jersey Supreme Court noted that the state had no important interest in compelling Quinlan to "endure the unendurable, only to vegetate a few measurable months with no realistic possibility of returning to any semblance of cognitive or sapient life" (*In re Quinlan* 1976). The court's use of the language of "vegetate" and the assumption of the loss of "cognitive or sapient life" indicate how rapidly and thoroughly the common perception of the persistent VS took hold at the time, and how quickly it was integrated into jurisprudence. The court considered Quinlan's condition to be "debilitated and moribund" and "cruel and most unusual."

Those views were echoed 14 years later by the United States Supreme Court in the Nancy Cruzan case. In 1983, Cruzan, then 25 years old, was ejected from her car in a crash. She landed face down in a watery ditch. When found by paramedics, she had no vital signs, but she was resuscitated. She experienced an extended interval of anoxia and was comatose for 3 weeks, and then was diagnosed in a PVS. Five years later, her family sought to have artificial nutrition and hydration (ANH) withdrawn. Because most VS patients are not dependent on a ventilator, withdrawing ANH is often the only legally available way to hasten death for these individuals. In the Court's majority opinion, Justice John Paul Stevens contemplated the quality of life of the VS patient: "If she has any awareness of her surroundings, her life must be a living hell" (*Cruzan v. Director, Missouri Department of Health* 1990). He went

---

[8] Quinlan unexpectedly survived the removal of the ventilator. Like most VS patients, she was able to breathe on her own. She lived another 9 years before dying of pneumonia in 1985. After her death, an autopsy revealed extensive damage to her thalamus, providing early evidence of the role of the thalamus in consciousness (Kinney et al. 1994).

on to argue for the propriety of considering quality of life in right-to-die cases:

> It is appropriate to consider the quality of life in making decisions about the extraordinary medical treatment. Those who have made decisions about such matters without resort to the courts certainly consider the quality of life, and balance this against the unpleasant consequences to the patient. (*Cruzan v. Director, Missouri Department of Health* 1990)

There is evident and unresolved tension in the Supreme Court's ruling and in popular perceptions about quality of life in the VS. It appears to be commonly believed that quality of life is irremediably and inevitably bad in the VS, even though by definition the VS is a state of insensate unconsciousness in which the individual experiences no subjective states, good or bad. Justice Stevens' assertion that if Nancy Cruzan "has any awareness of her surroundings, her life must be a living hell" evinces a fundamental misunderstanding of what it means to be unconscious. There is clearly some other cryptic, value-laden meaning—something other than subjective well-being—attached to the phrase "quality of life" in such considerations of VS patients.

The Supreme Court did not rule in favor of Cruzan's family. In a 5 to 4 decision, the Court held that although competent individuals have the right to refuse medical treatment under the Due Process Clause, incompetent persons were not able to exercise such rights. They upheld Missouri's strict "clear and convincing" evidence standard for evaluating evidence of a patient's prior wishes and found the State of Missouri's actions designed to preserve human life to be constitutional. They sent the case back to the state courts. The Cruzans gathered more evidence that Nancy Cruzan would have wanted life support terminated, and when the State of Missouri withdrew from the case, a county probate judge ruled that the Cruzans had met the evidentiary standard. Nancy Cruzan's feeding tube was withdrawn on December 14, 1990, and she died 12 days later.[9]

Two years after the Cruzan decision, the British High Court, again echoing common sentiments, decided that ANH could be withdrawn from Tony Bland, a young man who was in a persistent VS after a being crushed in a stampede at a soccer match. The High Court concluded that "To his parents and family [Bland] is 'dead.' His spirit has left him and all that remains is the shell of his body" (Fergusson 1992). That ruling prompted Jennett to grant in a commentary the possibility of recovery from the PVS, which he noted would be more curse than blessing: "The recovery of a limited degree of awareness may indeed be worse than non-sentience for the patient" (Jennett 1992). Jennett praised the High Court for judging that it would be in Bland's best interests to have ANH withdrawn, noting again that the price of saving those patients with a "reasonable probability of meaningful recovery and of regaining life as a social person" is paid by "patients who die after a fruitless fight in intensive care or survive with irreparable brain damage" (Jennett 1992).

It is difficult to make sense of the claim that anything can be in an unconscious individual's current "best interests" if having interests at all requires consciousness. Likewise, it is difficult to reconcile the idea of unconsciousness and insentience with suffering or having a poor quality of life. Nonetheless, it is not uncommon for such claims to be made concerning these patients.

Reflecting on the swift certainty that prevailed in those early days, neurologist D. Alan Shewmon was critical of the "dogmatic assertions" that followed from a conflation of certainty about consciousness based on behavioral evidence and subsequent assumptions about brain anatomy. Those assertions, Shewmon argued,

---

[9] Six years later, in August 1996, Nancy Cruzan's father, Lester Cruzan, killed himself.

were based not on scientific evidence but on an unproved and philosophically biased assumption that consciousness is an "emergent property" of cortical neurons, at a time of intense socio-political pressure to provide courts with the medical "facts" about PVS. It is not the first time in history, and no doubt not the last, that one generation's medical "facts" become future generations' medical myths. (2004, 346)

Those dogmatic certainties persist. The right to die and DoCs have been entwined from the beginning, and it was the utter hopelessness of the persistent VS that inspired and gave fuel to those who fought for the legal right to "die with dignity," without medical interventions maintaining a life some view to be pointless, perhaps even worse than death. Indeed, when Jennett and Plum wrote of the persistent VS in 1972, it *was* a seemingly hopeless condition, an artifact of medical progress that saved many lives, but did so indiscriminately, without the capacity to distinguish those who would go on to recover and those who would remain forever trapped in an existence devoid of experience, social interaction, feeling, and thought. Decades on, it remains challenging to accurately predict recovery from brain injury and DoCs.

2.4 From Ethical Certainty to Uncertainty

Jennett and Plum described persistent VS patients as hopeless cases, "incapable of communication and without hope of recovery as social human beings." The "hopeful" cases, they said explicitly, are the ones who awaken from coma with signs of cortical functioning, unlike the persistent VS patients. In this description and designation of the persistent VS, the idea of *hopelessness* thus makes an early appearance, and Jennett and Plum were well aware of its ethical and social significance:

The immediate issue is to recognize that there is a group of patients who never show evidence of a working mind. . . . Certainly the indefinite survival of patients in this state presents a problem with humanitarian and socioeconomic implications which society as a whole will have to consider. If it were possible to predict soon after the brain damage had been sustained that, in the event of survival, the outcome would be a vegetative, mindless state, then the wisdom of continuing supportive measures could be discussed. (1972)

Thus, early in the history of the VS, ethical questions were raised—and seemingly answered—about whether life is worth living for these "mindless" patients, who were viewed as the unfortunate collateral damage of the effort to save the lives of those with severe brain injuries. Saving those who were not hopeless cases meant saving some who were, because outcomes could not be predicted.

That sense of hopelessness continues to be pervasive and persistent in both medical and bioethical discourses and practices. The VS has been called "a fate worse than death" (Feinberg and Ferry 1984), in which maintaining life support is a "futile endeavor" that cannot benefit the patient (Jennett and Dyer 1991). VS patients are frequently characterized as being as good as dead, such as in an account that appeared in a bioethics journal, describing a doctor in a VS as "lying in an open grave" (Crisci 1995). It has been argued that the permanent VS patient should be considered dead, because "the body in PVS has lost all forms of personhood" (Ravelingien et al. 2004). Jeff McMahan (1995) argued that individuals who have permanently lost the capacity for consciousness and mental activity are no longer living *persons* (although they may continue to be alive as human organisms). The humanity and personhood of VS patients has been frequently challenged on the grounds that "they permanently lack the most essential feature of the human being, which is its undisputed capacity for living the life of a person, or rational self-consciousness" (Rich 1997).

The view that the VS is a condition *worse than death* is also frequently endorsed by the public, with some attributing less mind to the vegetative patient than to the dead, and viewing them as "more dead than dead" (Gray, Knickman, and Wegner 2011).[10] Many family members of DoC patients view their loved ones as being in an ambiguous state—not straightforwardly alive, and not simply dead—cadavers with heartbeats.

Persons with DoCs thus remain exceptionally marginalized, set apart from the general population and from other people with brain injuries. Their ontological, diagnostic, and moral segregation has resulted in their contested personhood and moral status, challenges to their right to medical resources (Johnson 2010), and acceptance that the right to die is their only remaining right. DoCs reveal how conceptions of personhood or moral status that are contingent on consciousness are deeply vexed, given that unconsciousness is both liable to fluctuation and epistemically uncertain. Even if loss of personhood occurs only with the *permanent* loss of consciousness, it remains epistemically flimsy and requires admitting that we are at present wrong about 40 percent of the time about who is not a person.

2.5 What's in a Name?

Whatever the intended original meaning, the term *vegetative state* today functions as a "thick concept." Thick concepts are those that are not merely *descriptive,* but are also laden with *evaluative* and *normative* meaning and import. The idea of thick concepts comes

---

[10] There may well be cultural variation in those perceptions. A study by Inga Steppacher and Johanna Kissler found that Germans are significantly less negative in their assessments of patients in the VS/UWS than Americans (Steppacher and Kissler 2018). Importantly, Germans viewed VS/UWS patients as having minds and rejected the idea that VS/UWS is equivalent to, or less than, death. In Japan, the public and physicians alike tend not to view VS patients as persons, but also reject withdrawal of LST (Asai et al. 1999; Bito and Asai 2007).

from Bernard Williams, who distinguished them from "thin" evaluative concepts like "bad" and "good" (Williams 2011).[11] Thick concepts, by contrast, are descriptive—they describe something. But they also have evaluative or normative content—they have positive or negative ethical valence.[12] *Vegetative* is a description of the syndrome, one in which the "vegetative" or basic biological functions of a living organism continue, while the rational, cognitive, sapient functions have ceased. In common usage, however, it has taken on a pejorative meaning, owing no doubt to the conflation with *vegetable*. To speakers unfamiliar with its archaic meaning, *vegetative* implies *vegetable-like*. A concept like "vegetable" isn't obviously thick in its common usage, but applied to a human, it is thickened, and implies a less-than-human status. As a diagnosis and prognosis, even stripped of the prefixes *persistent* and *permanent*, "vegetative state" portends a life without value, meaning, or humanity, and in practice has *prescriptive* implications:

> "Vegetative" is not a purely descriptive definition. . . . It carries dehumanizing connotations, and since for the majority of people it is associated with a life not worth living, it may serve as a heuristic (intentionally or not) to steer decision-making toward WOLST [withdrawal of life-sustaining treatment]. (Lazaridis 2019)

Vegetative is not unique among medical terms in becoming thickened by common understanding in a way not intended. Terms like *moron* and *idiot* were in the early 20th century used descriptively in psychology to label specific levels of intellectual disability,

---

[11] To my knowledge, Christos Lazaridis was the first to describe *vegetative* in terms of Williams' thick concepts (Lazaridis 2019).

[12] An example of a thick concept is "selfish." Merriam-Webster's dictionary defines it as: "concerned excessively or exclusively with oneself: seeking or concentrating on one's own advantage, pleasure, or well-being without regard for others." That's a descriptive definition, but "selfish" is also a thick concept with evaluative or normative meaning—selfishness is usually thought to be a morally bad trait.

having an IQ of 51–70 and 0–25, respectively. The terms fell out of use and were retired from the medical lexicon (along with others like *imbecile* and *feeble-minded*) as they took on overwhelmingly negative, stigmatized connotations and were commonly used as insults.[13] To call someone an "idiot" might be in some sense descriptive—it might describe behaviors that are imprudent or ill-informed—but it is unmistakably an evaluative or normative claim, an insult, as well.

One of the motives for adopting UWS as an alternative to VS was to avoid the pejorative connotations and stigma associated with *vegetative*. *Unresponsive* and *wakeful* are thin, descriptive terms—they describe the observable behaviors of patients with the syndrome and don't have evaluative or normative meaning. UWS also recognizes the diagnostic and prognostic uncertainty of unconsciousness through its emphasis on describing patients as unresponsive and thereby remaining agnostic regarding consciousness (Laureys et al. 2010). Thinning of medical terminology to weed out stigmatizing terms and phrases sometimes follows changes in societal perceptions and usages, but it can also, importantly, drive those changes in ways that can benefit affected persons. Given the profoundly dehumanizing connotations of the term *vegetative*, a shift in terminology has the potential to help reframe both medical and ethical discourses in a way that is more responsive to the current understanding of the disorder and of patients. "Vegetative" is not commonly used as an insult, but it nonetheless has negative evaluative meaning and has become quite stigmatized in a way that harms DoC patients whose moral status, personhood, and right to treatment are frequently

---

[13] An example of legal assimilation of such terms can be found in Oliver Wendell Holmes' infamous statement in the 1927 Supreme Court decision *Buck v. Bell* upholding the legality of eugenicist sterilization of so-called "feeble-minded" women: "Three generations of imbeciles are enough." This shows how stigmatizing medical language is dehumanizing and harmful.

contested. I rather doubt it can be rehabilitated, any more than "idiot" can be.[14]

With all its medical, scientific, legal, and ethical baggage, *vegetative* should be retired as a diagnostic/prognostic entity, in favor of a thinner, descriptive, neutral term that recognizes the uncertainty of consciousness and unconsciousness. Perhaps UWS will be that term, although to date there has been limited uptake of UWS outside of Europe. In the neuroscientific, medical, and bioethical literature it is often paired with VS, which may do as a transitional measure, although some of the benefits will be lost if the baggage follows the phrase.

2.6 By Any Other Name

Taxonomic discussions have been a part of DoC history since the beginning—and there is ongoing debate about whether the current names and categories are sufficient to capture the subtlety, diversity, and variety of these disorders and the people who have them. Interest in revisiting the DoC taxonomy, both for reasons of scientific accuracy, and because of the ethical implications of the labels currently used, has increased in recent years, parallel to the growth in knowledge.

While it is commonly said that no two DoC patients are alike, owing to the great variety of brain injuries involved, there are only four fundamental categories for DoCs—two for unconscious states, and two for conscious states, with only the MCS subcategorized into different levels of functioning. (CMD, as mentioned above,

[14] Another medical term, *vegetation*, refers to abnormal growths of valvular tissues in infective endocarditis. The growths, which are collections of microbes, platelets, and fibrin, are so called because of their plant-like or fungus-like appearance. This use of *vegetation* is strictly descriptive, but it's worth noting that this medical usage of *vegetation* describes the visual resemblance to actual vegetation. *Vegetative* is commonly although metaphorically understood to describe a resemblance to the cognitive capacities of a plant.

spans categories.) Are these four categories sufficient to describe and categorize the complexity, diversity, and variety of impairment and functioning found in DoC patients, or do they obscure more than they clarify?

Changes in terminology and classification often follow enhanced understanding of disorders and disease mechanisms, and there have been several such changes since Jennett and Plum first named and described the persistent VS, including the adoption of *permanent* VS two decades later to recognize temporal boundaries for a change in prognosis. It was three decades before diagnostic criteria for the MCS were formally defined (Giacino et al. 2002). At the time, James Bernat, pondering the newly named MCS, wondered how well it tracked consciousness rather than responsiveness, although his concern was that we could not be sure that a patient had only "minimal" awareness, and not more.

> At the bedside, one can only crudely measure evidence of the fullness of human awareness. So how can we be certain that the awareness of patients in MCS is minimal? Given that the criteria for MCS measure impaired responsiveness, perhaps it would be more accurate to use the older term "minimally responsive" to describe them. (2002b)

Bernat's concerns about the MCS were well founded. Something like these concerns motivated the proposal to change the VS to UWS 10 years later.

Change began to accelerate. In 2006, the first cases of covertly aware patients were reported, and in 2009, 7 years after the MCS was defined, the subcategorization into MCS+/- was proposed (Gosseries et al. 2011), marking the differences in behavioral responsiveness Bernat flagged years earlier. A year after that, the European Task Force proposed changing the name of the VS to UWS. Nine years after the first covertly aware patients were identified, CMD was coined (Schiff 2015), replacing the placeholder name *functionally locked-in* (which risked confusion with locked-in syndrome, a brain disorder that is not a DoC).

More radical reforms of the entire taxonomy of DoCs have been proposed, acknowledging that the behaviorally defined categories fail to capture the differences in *consciousness* that are of scientific and ethical interest (Bayne, Hohwy, and Owen 2017). Lionel Naccache has proposed changing the MCS to cortically mediated state (CMS), reflecting the presence of behaviors that are complex and cortically generated. Naccache has also proposed eight categories of DoCs, which include distinctions based on the source of evidence (e.g., behavioral, neuroimaging) used to define the clinical state (Naccache 2017). In sketching possible categories, Naccache retained two categories each of coma and VS/UWS. Like Bayne et al., Naccache noted the incongruity inherent in inferring subjective mental states from objective, nonmental behaviors. But Naccache further argued that the MCS covers

[a] large and heterogeneous set of states that may span from unconscious patients with residual islets of cortical activity that translates into overt behavior, to conscious but cognitively impaired patients that may be self-conscious but unable to go from preserved response to command to the functional use of a communication code, due to executive deficits (working memory, executive control). (2017)

If that's right, then "minimally conscious" is a misnomer (as Bernat suggested), for MCS includes both conscious and unconscious individuals who exhibit cognitively mediated behavior. Naccache noted that this conclusion tracks with the distinction between MCS- patients who exhibit "cognitively poor" behaviors like visual fixation and pursuit, and MCS+ patients who show "cognitively richer" behaviors like reliable responses to verbal commands.

Concerns about the taxonomy of DoCs, and the names of DoCs, are not mere side discussions by fussy academics. Revising and

standardizing the language used for DoCs serve important ontological, epistemic, and ethical purposes. How DoCs are described
and what we call them should, at minimum, describe reality. Ideally,
we want our ontology to carve nature at its joints, to borrow Plato's
metaphor, so our classifications identify actual distinctions and
entities. Terminology that more accurately describes the changing
and mercurial clinical picture of DoCs would benefit from knocking
down the monoliths of *conscious* and *unconscious*. A multidimensional taxonomy that includes clinically and ethically meaningful
behavioral and cognitive capacities, etiology, time and chronicity,
diagnostic/assessment methodologies, and the subtleties of neural
function and dysfunction would add needed and informative nu-
ance and understanding to clinical diagnosis and prognosis, and to
on-the-ground decision-making on behalf of patients.

A rationally justified revision and standardization of the language used to represent these disorders should avoid already thick
concepts.[15] After decades of use and misuse, the term *vegetative* is
stigmatized, frequently misunderstood, and loaded with negative
meaning for patients, surrogates, and medical staff, and the *minimal* in minimally conscious state is close to having a similar fate.
Thus any effort to refine or expand the taxonomy of DoCs should
be attentive to the need for less fraught and suggestive terminology
that more accurately describes the changing and changeable clinical picture of DoCs (Lazaridis, Desai, and Johnson 2021). We also
need a taxonomic ethics—one that governs how we talk about these
patients and their disorders, and that includes what we call these
disorders, and consequently, what we call these patients.

---

[15] Whether it is possible to invent terms that are resistant to thickening is another
issue, given the constant evolution of meaning and connotation in language. The use of
geographical names for viruses is an example. While descriptive in the sense that they
are meant to describe the first known origin of a virus, such as Ebola virus, the association with a place can be stigmatizing (or used for propaganda and incitement, such as
attaching names like "Wuhan Flu" and "Chinese Virus" to SARS-CoV-2).

2.7 "Progress is the mother of problems"

—G. K. Chesterton

For decades, certainty prevailed concerning DoCs. Affected individuals were considered beyond treatment and beyond hope of recovery. They were considered to be nonpersons, even dead. Ethical debate almost exclusively focused on the value or disvalue of continued existence, whether these patients might be better off dead, and the permissibility of hastening death through the withdrawal of life-sustaining treatment (LST).

The erosion of certainty about DoCs began slowly, as a trickle of knowledge that first refined and expanded the diagnostic categories. New research and information have rapidly altered the medical and neuroscientific landscape, as well as the moral landscape, presenting new and pressing social, ethical, and legal challenges.

The science of DoCs has moved from an age of nihilism and hopelessness to an age of discovery. At the same time, new uncertainties about these disorders, and patients, have grown, thus ushering in an age of uncertainty. Corresponding advances in the social, legal, and ethical discourses about DoCs have been slow to follow these discoveries and to reckon with the new uncertainty. Where *ethical* certainty once prevailed, such certainty is unfounded while *epistemic* uncertainty persists. Or so I argue in the chapters to come.

3

Uncertainty

*Thus the unfacts, did we possess them, are too imprecisely
few to warrant our certitude . . .*
—James Joyce, *Finnegans Wake*, p. 57

It seems intuitively a bad thing when medical uncertainty about a
disease or disorder increases. We like to have more certainty with
our progress, thank you very much. We want more accurate diagnosis and prognosis and a clear understanding of etiology, disease
mechanisms, and progression. That is not, of course, how it always
works. Seemingly plausible theories and understandings about
disease, disorder, and illness are supplanted by other plausible
theories and understandings. Some move us closer to the truth,
and some do not. Importantly, it is not unusual for advances and
increases in knowledge to raise new scientific questions and to result in new and urgent ethical and social dilemmas. Advances can
both muddle and clarify.

The relatively brief history of disorders of consciousness (DoCs)
has seen two epistemic eras—the first was marked by certainty,
both ethical and epistemic, about the persistent vegetative state
(PVS). The second era has been notable for its epistemic and ethical
uncertainty, as new discoveries and new understanding of these
disorders have made more urgent long-standing concerns about
misdiagnosis as well as concerns about our ethical obligations to
patients with DoCs. Replacing certainty with uncertainty does not
sound like progress, but the current age of uncertainty presents

opportunities to reconsider, with epistemic humility, the dogmas engendered by the false hopelessness and certainties of the past. They were well-meaning certainties, and hopelessness was not a product of bad will or bad faith, but of epistemic limitations colliding with the mystery of consciousness. The ethical and social effects—the marginalization, neglect, and dehumanization of DoC patients, their contested personhood and contested right to life-sustaining treatment—can and must be addressed by attending to both the fact of uncertainty and the ethical obligations that follow from it.

Consider the history of Trisomy 21 (T21), or Down syndrome. In the 19th and 20th centuries, doctors and scientists sought to understand the cause of what was once called "mongolism" (a reference to the distinctive phenotypic appearance of the eyes of persons with T21). To modern sensibilities, the early writing, with references to "Mongolian idiots," is horrifying. John Langdon Down, namesake of Down syndrome, in his book *Observations on an Ethnic Classification of Idiots* (1866), thought T21 represented a racial "retrogression" caused by "instances of degeneracy arising from tuberculosis in the parents" (quoted in Patterson and Costa 2005). Various causes were considered in the decades that followed: degeneracy, syphilis, alcoholism, consanguinity, and uterine exhaustion, to name a few. R. L. Jenkins, reviewing what was known about "mongolism" in 1933, suggested several maternal causes, including "pathological change in the uterine mucosa," "toxic action of the secretions of the female generative tract," and "diminished viability of the ova," the last of which he thought the most likely (Jenkins 1933).[1]

---

[1] Jenkins attempted to helpfully clarify the terminology then in use by explaining that "the term Mongolian idiot is . . . a misnomer, as most of the children are not idiots, but imbeciles; neither are they mongolian" (Jenkins 1933, 506). The terms *idiot* and *imbecile* did, in the early 20th century, have more or less technical meaning as psychological classifications of cognitive/intellectual disability. They have fortunately fallen entirely out of use as medical concepts.

A decade later, Theodore Ingalls hypothesized that "the condition originates between the sixth and ninth week of fetal life" (Ingalls 1947), based on then current knowledge of embryonic development. Despite nearly a century of study, they were all as wrong as wrong could be about T21. By the late 1950s it was understood that T21 results from a trisomy, or extra copy, of chromosome 21. In the decades since, average life expectancy for persons with T21 has improved, from less than 1 year to more than 60 years. Persons with T21 are no longer institutionalized in much of the world, but live at home with their families, are educated in inclusive school settings, have jobs, get married, and have families of their own. It is understood that there is a spectrum of intellectual and physical impairment in T21, and that persons with T21 frequently enjoy good quality of life. Progress. At the same time, progress in the development of prenatal diagnosis, including noninvasive and earlier prenatal diagnosis, has made it possible to detect T21 earlier in pregnancy, and at lower risk to the pregnancy. Some 90 percent of affected fetuses are terminated after prenatal diagnosis, a state of affairs that advocates and persons with T21 do not think represents ethical progress or appropriate acceptance and social inclusion of those with T21 (Kaposy 2013, 2018). Instead, it treats T21 as a problem best solved by preventing the birth and existence of people with T21.[2]

We are in much the same place with DoCs, as increased knowledge and understanding of these disorders have generated new scientific questions about them, but also new and more urgent ethical questions about DoC patients. Among the issues most in need of attention are the diagnostic, prognostic, and ethical uncertainties concerning DoCs.

---

[2] In the chapters to follow, I discuss the prevention of DoCs through withdrawal of LST. As is also true of T21, there is uncertainty about what a diagnosis/prognosis portends for persons with brain injuries, and at least one goal of early withdrawal of LST is the prevention of chronic DoCs and disability.

3.1 The Problem of Progress

When the PVS was first named and defined, there was medical certainty about the diagnosis and prognosis of unconsciousness. Ethical consensus quickly coalesced around a disorder considered untreatable and hopeless, and in which life could have no value. There emerged during this period growing concern about medical advancements that had unforeseen and unfortunate consequences, including the unwanted prolongation of life. Jennett and Plum presciently wondered about the wisdom of continuing life-sustaining treatment for "vegetative, mindless" patients, and predicted that "the indefinite survival in this state presents a problem with humanitarian and socioeconomic implications which society as a whole will have to consider" (Jennett and Plum 1972). Four years earlier, the Ad Hoc Committee of the Harvard Medical School to Examine the Definition of Brain Death published "A Definition of Irreversible Coma" (Beecher et al., 1968), inventing a new way of defining death to respond to a related problem created by improvements in intensive care: patients with severe neurological injuries and no hope of recovering consciousness who could be kept alive indefinitely. Lewis Thomas, around the same time, worried about the enormous costs of "halfway technologies," those

> things that must be done after the fact, in efforts to compensate
> for the incapacitating effects of certain diseases whose course one
> is unable to do very much about. It is a technology designed to
> make up for disease, or to postpone death. (1971)

Albert Jonsen, reflecting on medical innovation and the birth of bioethics in the 1960s and 1970s, noted that the ancient Hippocratic admonition to benefit the sick

> had become difficult to apply in the setting of modern medi-
> cine. The respiratory, renal, and cardiac technologies that had

come into being during the postwar era could produce wondrous physiological effects. It was not always clear, however, that those effects were benefits for the patients in whose body they were produced.... Prolongation of life is too simple a measure of benefit. (1993, S3)

Although the PVS had long been recognized under different names, its emergence into modern medicine and public awareness came at a time when doctors, the public, and the nascent discipline of bioethics were increasingly concerned about the ethical propriety of keeping people alive when they had little hope of "meaningful recovery," as well as concern about the potential social and financial costs. It was also a period when modern medicine in the West was transitioning from a paternalistic "doctor knows best" model of medicine to one that focused more on patient autonomy and rights. In the legal case of Karen Ann Quinlan, all those trend lines converged in an endorsement of a "right to die," conceived as a right against being kept alive when life was no longer desired or desirable. The idea that death is preferable to the PVS firmly took root, with both ethical and legal offshoots. The *Quinlan* and *Cruzan* cases set enduring legal precedents for the right of surrogates to decide to withdraw life-sustaining treatment (LST) on behalf of vegetative patients. The more expansive right-to-die debate concerning assisted suicide and Medical Aid in Dying (MAiD) for other patients continues. The precedents set by *Quinlan* and *Cruzan* apply narrowly to patients in the vegetative state/unresponsive wakefulness syndrome (VS/UWS). In the United States, many states have carved out exceptions for withdrawing LST from chronically unconscious patients, but not those with other DoCs or conditions, and decades on, extending MAiD to other persons remains largely contested and unresolved as both legal and ethical matters.

3.2 A Neuroscientific Revolution

In 1984, Terry Wallis, a 19-year-old Arkansan, was in a pickup truck that skidded off a bridge. The accident left him comatose, with a severely injured brain. He was eventually diagnosed as being in a PVS. He spent the next 19 years of his life in a nursing home. Family members who visited him reported seeing signs of awareness. Not possible, they were told. People don't recover from PVS.

On June 11, 2003, 19 years after his accident, Wallis spoke. He said "Mom." Researchers who scanned his brain later concluded that Wallis's brain, although still showing signs of damage and atrophy, had repaired itself, with evidence of axonal regrowth that continued after his "awakening," along with continued functional improvements in speech, cognition, and movement (Voss et al. 2006). Wallis, it was concluded, had been in a minimally conscious state (MCS) for most of those 19 years. MCS did not formally exist as a diagnostic category until 2002, the year before Wallis said "Mom." At the time of his initial diagnosis, there were only two DoCs: coma and the persistent VS.

Wallis now lives with his parents in their home. His mother Angilee Wallis recounts a family gathering where he spontaneously declared "Mama, life is good!" (in Fins 2015, 246).

3.2.1 Kate Bainbridge

Several years before Terry Wallis spoke, a 26-year-old British schoolteacher named Kate Bainbridge was diagnosed in a VS after contracting encephalomyelitis. She went to hospital in June 1997 with altered consciousness after several days of a sore throat and headaches. A CT scan revealed diffuse cerebral edema and acute disseminated encephalomyelopathy with large brain lesions in both thalami. She was in a VS or MCS for 5–6 months, during which time she could open her eyes but couldn't communicate and did not show evidence of responsiveness. Bainbridge then recovered consciousness, and her cognitive and emotional recovery over several years is well-documented in published papers (that credit her as a co-author). There are chilling details of the distress and pain she experienced when her caregivers thought she was unconscious:

> Well I was screaming as they caused me so much pain. I don't want any body to have the same awful time as I did. I think my case shows don't treat people as text book cases. (Kate Bainbridge, quoted in Wilson, Gracey, and Bainbridge 2001)

Bainbridge's experience highlights both the importance of getting the diagnosis right and the significant risks for misdiagnosed patients, who can endure pain, isolation, and emotional distress when being treated as if they are "not there."

> They treated me as if I was stupid in (hospital). My stay there was absolute hell they never told me anything. They used to suction me through my mouth and they never told me why or what it was called they have never told me about my trachy [tracheostomy tube]. I am lucky I am with it and have a good memory so I could work it out. I don't want them to do it to anyone else. They have learnt a lot from me already, but I think telling people what you are doing is very important. I can't tell you how frightening it was, especially suction through the mouth. I tried to hold my breath to get away from all the pain. They never told me about my tube. I wondered why I did not eat. (Kate Bainbridge in October 2000, quoted in Wilson, Gracey, and Bainbridge 2001)

Within a few years after her injury, Bainbridge's cognitive assessments showed her intellectual, executive, and memory skills within the normal range. She did not recover the ability to speak, which she found distressing:

> Not being able to talk is my biggest handicap; as people think I am out of it. I think it would be better if I was out of it so I would not get so upset so much. . . . Not being able to talk is very hard for me people think I am stupid and talk to me gently. (Kate Bainbridge in 2001, quoted in Wilson, Gracey, and Bainbridge 2001)

Her emotional recovery, also well-documented, was difficult, and she was traumatized by her experiences while hospitalized and in rehabilitation.

> Kate presented as withdrawn and depressed. She was prone to screaming, especially during physiotherapy, and was known to bite other people—often this would be when others would be helping with her personal care. From a behavioural perspective, Kate's behavior could be seen as a communication to those providing her care that she was frightened and in pain. Kate's difficulties with communication and her reliance upon a communication board often resulted in frustration for her and her carers, as misunderstandings would be common. (Macniven et al. 2003)

> Everyone thinks they [the hospital staff] are good, but even my medical care got worse and worse. I think they are useless except in intensive care . . . I thought they just enjoyed hurting me [during suction] and scaring me as they took no notice of my screams. Can you see how angry I am? In my last illness I got a collapsed lung and pneumonia, it was their fault. (Kate Bainbridge, quoted in Macniven et al. 2003)

Before her illness, Bainbridge had been engaged to be married and was hoping to have "lots" of children. She was described by her family as "very bright, kind, shy, and quiet," a young woman with a happy life who had been thinking about her future. Macniven et al. documented how Bainbridge's emotional recovery and adjustment had been neglected until cognitive assessments revealed that she was "functioning at a much higher level than people had assumed." Her emotional recovery was aided by cognitive therapy and anger management techniques.

> I can't believe how much I have changed . . . I now want to be alive and I am looking forward to the future. . . . I can now keep myself occupied and busy, instead of sitting on my own doing nothing . . . I just don't want anyone else to have such an awful time as me. I can now see it is over and hopefully I will never have it again . . . Can you see how angry I used to feel, but now there is no point in being angry, I just need to look to the future. (Kate Bainbridge, quoted in Macniven et al. 2003)

Bainbridge is also the first documented case of what is now called cognitive motor dissociation (CMD)—a patient who met diagnostic criteria for VS but exhibited specific and identifiable brain activations in response to a stimulus. Four months after her illness, neuroscientist Adrian Owen and colleagues put her in a PET scanner and showed her photographs of faces, some belonging to her family members and some distorted and unrecognizable. When images of her family appeared, Bainbridge's brain showed activations of the fusiform gyrus, an area of the brain correlated with facial recognition (Menon et al. 1998). The activations were identical to those seen in the brains of healthy volunteers. (It is unclear if Bainbridge was in a VS or MCS at the time. Menon et al. reported that she was in a VS, while Wilson et al. reported that Bainbridge claimed to remember things from that time period, which is also when she began screaming at staff. CMD, however, spans DoC categories, and the important point here is that Bainbridge was not behaviorally responsive in a way that indicated she had the cognitive capacities or awareness to perform the mental tasks inferred from the PET scan responses.)

3.2.2 Behaving Brains

Several years later, in 2006, Owen and colleagues published the results of an even more extraordinary experiment in which a patient, a 23-year-old woman diagnosed in a VS after a traumatic brain injury (TBI), was asked to perform two distinct, active mental imagery tasks: to imagine that she was playing a game of tennis, and to imagine that she was walking through the rooms of her home. In this experiment, during each imagery task, activations of the supplementary motor area (SMA), and of the parahippocampal gyrus, posterior parietal lobe, and lateral premotor cortex, respectively, could be seen using functional magnetic resonance imaging (fMRI).[3] The VS patient's brain activations were similar to those of healthy controls, indicating appropriate responses to being asked to perform the mental tasks. They showed that she was conscious and able to understand spoken commands (Owen et al. 2006).

Four years later, in a study of 54 patients diagnosed in the VS and MCS, five patients were able to "willfully modulate their brain activity" using the same tasks used in the Owen study. Four of the five were diagnosed in the VS. Of those four, subsequent bedside behavioral examination of two of them revealed some evidence of behavioral responsiveness (indicating misdiagnosis), while the other two showed no evidence of responsiveness or awareness (indicating that they met diagnostic criteria for VS). One patient, a young man with a TBI who had been diagnosed in a VS for 5 years, was able to communicate, answering autobiographical questions using the

---

[3] fMRI images show blood-oxygen-level-dependent (BOLD) signals in the brain. Essentially, BOLD shows areas of the brain where oxygen is being recruited, indicating activity. It does not show the mental activity itself—it is not literal mind reading, and there is no image of "imagine a game of tennis." Rather, it must be inferred from the BOLD signal that the area of the brain that "lights up" is being used. When the area is correlated with specific types of mental activity (e.g., navigation, facial recognition), it can be further inferred that the target mental activity is occurring. The experiments by Owen, Monti, and others first mapped and averaged BOLD signals in the areas of interest in healthy volunteers' typically functioning brains, then compared those maps to the activations in the experimental subjects.

same mental imagery tasks to indicate yes/no responses (Monti et al. 2010). None of these patients would have been able to perform these cognitive tasks if they were truly in a VS. That they could is evidence that they were not only aware, but retained cognitive capacities, including memory, imagination, language comprehension, and communication. The distinctive feature of CMD is that CMD patients are conscious and have cognitive capacities—such as the ability to understand spoken commands and perform mental tasks—that can at present be detected only using active neuroimaging paradigms such as fMRI. There is now abundant evidence that the brain that appears "vegetative" can retain several high-level cognitive functions, across sensory modalities, including language processing and learning dynamics (Monti 2012) and capacities like the ability to follow the plot of a movie (Naci et al. 2014). CMD patients also have capacities for pain, emotion processing, and recognizing familiar voices (Schnakers et al. 2012; Schnakers and Zasler 2007; Bekinschtein et al. 2004). As the experience of Kate Bainbridge makes painfully clear, neglecting or underestimating these capacities can have devastating physical, emotional, and psychological effects on patients.

CMD patients are *all* misdiagnosed as unconscious or minimally conscious, despite satisfying diagnostic criteria. This points to two important and related epistemic problems: first, the persistent problem of misdiagnosis, and second, the mismatch between the behavioral diagnosis of DoCs, and the thing—consciousness—being diagnosed. That mismatch is especially obvious in CMD patients who meet the diagnostic criteria for VS/UWS.

3.2.3 The Epistemic Limits of Behavioral Evidence

Localized injuries to the brain can result in specific deficits. For example, Broca's and Wernicke's aphasias result from damage to the "language areas" of the brain, respectively, and are often caused by stroke. These aphasias result in distinctively different language deficits that can be diagnosed behaviorally—Wernicke's aphasia causes affected patients to speak in long, nonsensical sentences, for example. But consciousness is not confined to a single area or structure of the brain, and it likely involves a network of functioning and complex signaling between areas of the brain. Although behavioral deficits in DoCs may be distributed, consciousness may be intact or present, as occurs in locked-in syndrome (with near total absence of behavior) and CMD. Thus, a fundamental question about the taxonomy of DoCs is why brain disorders that involve impairments of consciousness should be classified by outward manifestations of behaviors that crudely and unreliably capture differences in an individual's capacities for conscious experience.

The JFK Coma Recovery Scale–Revised (CRS-R) is an important behavioral test used for diagnosing impairments of, and recovery of, consciousness. The CRS-R contains six subscales addressing auditory, visual, motor, oromotor, communication, and arousal processes and associated behaviors. Some of these behaviors allow for strong inferences of consciousness, such as intelligible verbalization, functional object use, and object localization (reaching for an object).[4] Other behaviors (and behavioral unresponsiveness) are consistent with unconscious states, such as eye opening with or without stimulation, in the arousal subscale of the CRS-R. Two of the tests in the visual subscale involve visual fixation and visual pursuit, or the ability to fix one's gaze on an object and

[4] Functional object use (such as tool use) and object localization are widespread among animals, including insects, with tool use frequently taken to indicate intelligence and consciousness. There remain skeptics about animal consciousness who maintain that an animal might be conscious of a percept—of perceiving an object or event—without having mental states (like thoughts or beliefs) about it. Or animals might have unconscious percepts, interacting with their environments like sleepwalking humans (Carruthers 2018). If this view is correct, the implication is that functional object use and object localization do not require consciousness in humans either. And this might be correct. Sleepwalkers are able to engage in complex behaviors that include object localization and use. This raises interesting and important questions about what kind of conscious state such behaviors might require, and whether it is the sort of consciousness—global consciousness—we think is impaired in DoCs.

follow it with one's eyes. Visual fixation and pursuit are considered
behaviors indicative of consciousness and (minimally) the MCS diagnosis. Failure to detect fixation and pursuit has been associated
with misdiagnosis of VS/UWS in patients who were in the MCS.
A Dutch study found that 39 percent of patients reported as in the
VS/UWS were misdiagnosed and at least in the MCS, and visual
fixation and/or visual pursuit was undetected in more than half of
those in the study (Schnakers et al. 2009). A study by Andrews et al.
in 1996 found that 43 percent of patients in a neurorehabilitation
unit were misdiagnosed as being in the VS, and of those, 65 percent
were either blind or severely visually impaired, making their visual
nonresponsiveness liable to misinterpretation (Andrews et al.
1996). It remains a matter of debate whether visual fixation and
pursuit are reliable signs of consciousness (Overbeek et al. 2018).
Sensory deficits, such as cortical blindness or deafness, motor
impairments that limit movement and control of movement, and
language impairments like aphasia and apraxia after brain injuries
can all thwart behavioral assessment of consciousness and contribute to DoCs being so frequently misdiagnosed. Importantly, the
poor specificity of behavioral tests—how accurately they identify
unconscious individuals—is not attributable to the tester, but to the
tests themselves. Behavioral tests don't and can't directly test for the
target disorder (unconsciousness). Rather, the presence or absence
of consciousness must be inferred from the behavioral responsiveness or unresponsiveness of the patient.

Martin M. Monti and Adrian Owen have referred to "behavior
in the brain" as nonmotoric but voluntary behavior, and they argue
that "if observation of voluntary motor behavior can be taken as evidence of a state of awareness, observation of its underlying (voluntary) brain activity must also lead to the same conclusion" (Monti
and Owen 2010). This line of reasoning would extend the behavioral repertoire used in diagnosis of DoCs, and might go some way
toward reducing the number of misdiagnoses, although it remains
the case that some of the same confounds that can limit outward

behavioral responses can affect brain behaviors as well. Bayne et al. similarly argued that the evidential status of covert measures of consciousness—such as mental task command-following—can be justified by "appealing to the fact that they are direct analogues of currently accepted behavioral measures, and thus they inherit the evidential force of those behavioral measures" (Bayne, Hohwy, and Owen 2017, 869). And, like motoric behavioral unresponsiveness, negative "brain behavior" results are not dispositive—an absence of evident brain responsiveness is not evidence of the absence of consciousness. The low evidential, epistemic value of motoric behavioral responsiveness is, of course, precisely the problem that neuroimaging paradigms to detect covert consciousness hope to mitigate. That brain behaviors are still proxies of consciousness that require inferences should not temper enthusiasm for neurodiagnostic innovations, but neither should we think we have solved the misdiagnosis problem.

Consider aphasia again. Disordered speech is the sentinel symptom of aphasia, but aphasia is itself a symptom of a brain pathology, like a stroke or a brain tumor that lesions the Broca's or Wernicke's areas of the brain. We could say that aphasia as a disorder is a proxy for an injury or pathology that affects particular brain regions. Disordered consciousness, similarly, is a symptom of diverse brain injuries with a range of severity. Mild TBI, or concussions, can result in temporary loss of consciousness, and devastating brain injuries from a variety of causes, including localized TBIs and anoxic insults that cause global brain injury, can result in prolonged impairments of consciousness. In other words, there is really no natural kind that is *a* disorder of consciousness—DoCs are symptoms, and may be as diverse as the brain injuries of which they are symptoms. The specific encephalopathy can be important for both diagnostic and prognostic purposes, but behavioral proxies of unconsciousness are two steps removed from that. This makes it all the more difficult to diagnose and prognosticate about DoCs.

The current diagnostic categories for DoCs are coarse-grained. There are but four DoCs, despite considerable variation in the type, extent, and location of injury to the brain: coma, VS/UWS, MCS+/MCS-, and emergence from the MCS (EMCS). It is known that etiology makes a difference in outcomes. VS/UWS patients with TBI tend to have better outcomes than those with anoxic/hypoxic/ischemic brain injuries. Progressive neurodegenerative disorders like Alzheimer's dementia or Tay-Sachs disease can only be expected to get worse. The current taxonomy of DoCs does not reflect the prognostic significance of differences in etiology. Finer-grained distinctions are needed.

Depending on how granular we get, finer-grained diagnostic and prognostic categories might multiply considerably, much like the general category of cancer includes more than 100 specific types with different genetic, diagnostic, prognostic, and treatment profiles that include the location, cell type, and extent of metastasis. The grains in a finer-grained taxonomy of DoCs might also serve distinct diagnostic, prognostic, therapeutic, and ethical functions. No current diagnostic batteries can definitively identify DoCs or accurately prognosticate for individual patients, and it is especially challenging to do so in the early days following brain injury. As is discussed in the chapters to follow, diagnostic and prognostic uncertainty in the acute phase of brain injury is a significant epistemic problem in neurointensive care, and it is a locus of considerable ethical uncertainty, difficulty, and distress for surrogates faced with decision-making for injured and incapacitated patients.

The nature of the decisions that must be made concerning patients with DoCs is one reason that finer-grained distinctions are valuable and needed. But fixing solely on one feature of these disorders—that they appear to result in an impairment or loss of consciousness (or look that way behaviorally)—sees the forest but misses the trees.

3.3 Subtle Distinctions: Brain Death and the VS/UWS

Death by neurological criteria (DNC), known more commonly as brain death, is legally defined as death in numerous jurisdictions. In the United States, where the current legal standard is whole brain death, brain death is defined as the irreversible loss of all functions of the entire brain, including the brainstem. In practice, the tests used to determine brain death involve confirming the absence of brainstem reflexes, including gag, pupillary, and respiratory reflexes, and the absence of consciousness. Cortical electrical activity, hormonal function, and intracranial blood flow are all compatible with whole brain death as it is determined in practice. That is, the current diagnostic guidelines do not align with the statutory definition of whole brain death.

In the United Kingdom, a brainstem death standard is used. The reticular activating system and the nuclei for cardiorespiratory regulation reside in the brainstem and are key components of consciousness and respiratory control. Their functional destruction results in brainstem death.

> Death entails the irreversible loss of those essential characteristics which are necessary to the existence of a living human person . . . and thus, the definition of death should be regarded as the irreversible loss of the capacity for consciousness, combined with the irreversible loss of the capacity to breathe. (Academy of Medical Royal Colleges 2008)

The UK standard is clear about what is being diagnosed, and it is also clear about the justification—brain death is the death of the *person*. It explicitly claims that an essential feature of brain death is a loss of consciousness, and the other is apnea, when both are considered irreversible. The brain dead individual, unlike many in the VS/UWS, has lost the ability to breathe without a ventilator owing to damage to the brainstem. The Ad Hoc Committee of the Harvard Medical School to Examine the Definition of Brain Death, in setting out a definition of brain death in 1968, called it "irreversible coma," suggesting continuity, if not identity, with DoCs (Beecher et al. 1968). One might rightly ask if the only difference between brain death and coma is "irreversibility," or the lost potential for recovery. Because brain death is considered death, there is virtually no question that LST will be withdrawn, except in rare cases when a family or surrogate objects. (When the patient is an organ donor, LST is maintained temporarily to preserve the viability of their organs.[5]) That is, brain death with rare exceptions leads to death, full stop, because LST is withdrawn.

To date, there has been one documented case of possible recovery from DNC, and it is controversial. Jahi McMath was 13 years old when she had a tonsillectomy to treat sleep apnea, at an Oakland, California, hospital. She developed postsurgical bleeding that, according to her family, was ignored by the medical staff. Jahi experienced an hypoxic brain injury and was subsequently diagnosed as brain dead. Her mother, Nailah Winkfield, contested the DNC declaration, and a weeks-long legal battle followed. Jahi was eventually released to her mother, and was airlifted to New Jersey, where the law requires accommodation for those who reject DNC on religious grounds (Johnson 2016a). New Jersey's statute explicitly prohibits declarations of DNC under such circumstances and requires a declaration of death according to the circulatory-respiratory standard.

Jahi survived for four and a half years, cared for by her family in their home. Shewmon has argued that Jahi met the criteria for the MCS several months after she was diagnosed as brain dead

[5] I was once taken to task for referring to medical intervention that maintains the body in brain death as "life-sustaining treatment." Perhaps my interlocutor thought it provocative and tendentious. They argued that "physiological support," which doesn't imply that the patient is alive, was more accurate. It is also referred to as "organ support," although I think that is, in its dehumanizing employment of synecdoche, tendentious and offensive.

(Shewmon 2018). Importantly, Shewmon does not claim that Jahi was initially misdiagnosed. She met the accepted criteria for DNC. Rather, she might be the first known case of recovery in someone meeting the clinical criteria for DNC. If this is true, then by definition Jahi was not brain dead, as DNC includes an irreversibility criterion. Her case points to the problem of self-fulfilling prophecies, which is especially acute in neurology. The criteria for DNC include apneic coma in which the patient cannot breathe on their own, and so the withdrawal of LST (or physiological support, if you prefer) will result in death according to circulatory-respiratory criteria in short order. There have been documented cases of patients diagnosed as brain dead who spontaneously began breathing after withdrawal of the ventilator. By definition, they were misdiagnosed, but like misdiagnosis in DoCs, the culprits are the diagnostic criteria and confounding factors (Shewmon 2017; Latorre, Schmidt, and Greer 2020; Hansen and Joffe 2017). Since LST is almost always withdrawn after a diagnosis of brain death, it cannot be known how many potential misdiagnoses occur.

Critics of whole brain death have long argued that it is not truly equivalent to death, as somatic processes indicative of life continue when treatments like ventilatory support are maintained. These signs of life include growth, puberty, menstruation, wound healing, digestion, and even gestation of fetuses and childbirth. Moreover, it is argued, the diagnostic criteria used cannot ascertain that the entire brain has ceased functioning, per the definition, such that whole brain death is at best a misnomer, given the preservation of detectable brain activity.

Shewmon has long been skeptical of the criteria for DNC and has documented numerous "chronic" brain deaths, patients who were maintained for months or years after diagnosis (Shewmon 1998), providing evidence that the brain is not, in fact, necessary for the survival and functioning of the body. Shewmon argues that the criteria for brain death do not actually diagnose what they purport to diagnose, which is the irreversible cessation of all functions of the entire brain. Indeed, it's not clear why criteria like the loss of pupillary reflex (which is also absent in some blind persons) or the loss of spontaneous respiration signify death. Just as behavioral criteria for diagnosing unconsciousness don't actually capture unconsciousness, the criteria for brain death do not capture death.

Defenders of the whole brain death standard argue that what is critical is that whole brain death entails the "permanent cessation of the critical functions" of the brain, notwithstanding islands of functioning brain tissue and minimal brain activity (Bernat 1998). The definition of whole brain death equates bodily or biological death and neurological death by underscoring the role of the brain in "integrating" the somatic functions of living organisms. This is demonstrably untrue, however. Jahi McMath was in generally good health for most of her existence following the diagnosis of brain death.

In 2008, the President's Council on Bioethics provided a rationale for equating whole brain death and death, stating that "total brain failure can continue to serve as a criterion for declaring death . . . because it is a sign that this organism can no longer engage in the essential work that defines living things" (President's Council on Bioethics 2008). That essential work includes "self-preservation" and "need-driven commerce with the surrounding world." These, it was noted, require breathing and consciousness. Critics were quick to point to counterexamples of undeniably living humans who are unconscious and unable to breathe independently, including persons in apneic coma, high cervical quadriplegics in a VS/UWS, and fetuses (which can include fetuses being gestated by persons diagnosed as brain dead).

Circulatory-respiratory death is nearly universally accepted by cultures and spiritual traditions worldwide and is followed by rigor mortis and bodily decay—long understood to be indicators of death. Brain death is not as widely accepted, nor does it result in a decaying corpse. A philosophical underpinning of both whole brain death and brainstem death, however, is that the loss of brain function marks the death of a *person*, because it entails the irreversible loss of consciousness. Some philosophers and physicians have suggested an alternative to whole brain death and brainstem death, based on the understanding that whether the body or the brain can be said to have died or ceased functioning is beside the point. What matters, in their view, is that the *person* is dead and gone, whether or not the body or brain can still function. There are echoes here again of Aristotle's notion of the rational soul (as opposed to the nutritive/vegetative and sensitive soul) being a distinctly human capacity.

It is the permanent loss of consciousness, in this view, that is akin to death. Robert Veatch, for example, denied that death can be defined biologically, and argued for *moral* death: the loss of personhood is what is morally relevant, because it signals the loss of moral standing and appropriately precipitates death-related activities (Veatch 2005). Joseph Fletcher, a theologian and bioethicist, claimed that "the 'vegetable' patient, no matter how many spontaneous vital functions may be continuing, is dead, a nonperson" (Fletcher 1974, 7). Note that Fletcher referred to the person in the VS as a "vegetable" just 2 years after Jennett and Plum named the VS, a sign of the swiftness with which the conflation took hold even among those who should have known better than to call human beings "vegetables." McMahan argued that a human organism might be biologically alive, but "In many cases in which a patient enters a persistent vegetative state, what has happened is that the person has died or ceased to exist while the organism, sustained by the operations of the brainstem, remains alive" (McMahan 1995). The notion that the loss of consciousness is equivalent to the death of the person is something else brain death and the VS/UWS have in common.

Bernat, a defender of whole brain death, cautioned that if loss of consciousness is death, then people who are currently regarded as alive in every society and culture would be considered dead, and this "contrives a redefinition of death" (Bernat 2002a).

Problematically for the view that loss of consciousness is death is that there are individuals who have lost consciousness (perhaps permanently), such as those in the chronic VS/UWS, who are very much *not* considered dead yet, with all that death entails in the way of social, cultural, legal, and religious practices. We do not, for example, put them in a box and put them in the ground. If we declare VS/UWS patients to be not just metaphorically dead, or "as good as dead," but actually dead, then misdiagnosis in DoCs becomes an even more urgent problem, and one that would compound existing concerns about brain death as death (Johnson 2017a) and the diagnostic criteria for both DNC and DoCs. Given the epistemic uncertainty of loss of consciousness, let alone irreversible loss of consciousness, we would do well to remember Miracle Max's sage words, "There's a big difference between mostly dead and all dead. Mostly dead is slightly alive" (*The Princess Bride*).

3.4 After the Revolution: The Persistence of Diagnostic and Prognostic Uncertainty

3.4.1 Diagnostic Uncertainty

The problem of misdiagnosis in disorders of consciousness is well documented, has persisted for several decades (van Erp et al. 2015; Schnakers et al. 2009; Andrews et al. 1996), and is a major source of diagnostic uncertainty. The estimated rate of misdiagnosis— 39 to 43 percent—has resisted improvements in technology and neurointensive care, and awareness of the problem. Needless to say, when misdiagnosis occurs in four out of ten cases, there is cause for concern. It is cause for *alarm* when, as is the case with DoCs, a misdiagnosis can prompt treatment limitations or the withdrawal of LST.

Significant epistemic limitations are behind these very high rates of clinical misdiagnosis, and of particular note is the unreliability of the bedside clinical (behavioral) exam (Schnakers 2009). The mismatch between what is being tested (behavioral responsiveness) and what is being sought (a confirmation of consciousness) is part of the problem. Functional neuroimaging studies revealing the existence of covertly aware patients in CMD have shown that the initial understanding of VS patients as "mindless" (Jennett and Plum 1972) is surely inaccurate in at least a significant minority of patients. Neuroimaging, should it be validated and widely used in diagnosis, might reduce—but not eliminate—misdiagnosis. Nothing currently exists that can accurately diagnose every patient, given the diversity of injury and of functional and sensory loss. One can envision a future where we've identified the neural (or neuronal) correlates of consciousness (NCCs) and have high-resolution neuroimaging capabilities that might easily and quickly diagnose all manner of encephalopathies—a brain tricorder, as it were—but that future remains speculative and distant, and there are misdiagnosed patients, and others like Kate Bainbridge and Terry Wallis, now.

While there are interesting ontological questions about whether there is a bright line between consciousness and unconsciousness (Fischer and Truog 2017), I'm interested in the epistemic problems related to diagnosis and prognosis. We might think, of course, that if the ontological question is answered in the negative—there is no bright line between consciousness and unconsciousness—then looking for evidence of that line is fruitless, a quest with no endpoint. There is neurobiological support for some theories of consciousness, such as emergent property theories (Seth 2009; Edelman 1999) and the integrated information theory (Tononi et al. 2016), that suggest that consciousness(es) might exist along a continuum, rather than being an on/off phenomenon. If that is the case, then matters remain ontologically, diagnostically, and prognostically fuzzy, and ontological and ethical questions about appropriate thresholds will persist. All the ethical questions that are currently so vexing about DoC patients—*What is the moral significance of (various states/levels of) consciousness? What is owed to DoC patients? How ought we proceed ethically in the face of uncertainty?*—will remain vexing.

3.4.2 Prognostic Uncertainty

Faced with mortality, scientific knowledge can provide only an ounce of certainty: Yes, you will die. But one wants a full pound of certainty, and that is not on offer.
> —Paul Kalanithi in "How long have I got left?"

The epistemic problem of misdiagnosis in DoCs has long been recognized. Prognosis is secondary to diagnosis, so misdiagnosis can prompt prognostic pessimism, and treatment limitations and withdrawals that result in death. There is also potential for harm if patients—like Kate Bainbridge—experience avoidable pain and suffering due to unmet physical, emotional, and psychosocial needs.

The discovery of covertly conscious DoC patients has heightened concerns about prognostic uncertainty (Smith, White, and Arnold 2013; Johnson 2016a, 2016b). Case reports of late recoveries of patients, as well as long-term follow-up studies of chronic patients, have put in doubt the accepted time frames for considering DoCs stable and permanent (Steppacher, Kaps, and Kissler 2014, 2016; Kuehlmeyer et al. 2013), as well as the accuracy of current prognostic tools (Edlow et al. 2013). The prognostic uncertainty of the VS/UWS prompted the recommendation that the term *permanent* be removed from VS/UWS and that it be replaced with *chronic* (Giacino et al. 2018). Permanence is prognostic (and another thick concept laden with normative meaning), while chronic is descriptive, lacks the implication of impossibility, and is in harmony with wider medical usage. The way that "permanence" coupled with unconsciousness has been equated with death and nonpersonhood indicates how a word that in other contexts is benign can in this context be thick.

In the neurointensive care setting, where decisions are frequently made regarding the continuation, limitation, or withdrawal of treatment soon after brain injury, diagnostic and prognostic uncertainty raises important questions and doubts about decision-making concerning urgent matters of life and death (Turgeon et al. 2011; Côte et al. 2013; Hemphill and White 2009). The problem of the self-fulfilling prophecy and its contribution to outcomes across diverse etiologies of acute brain injury is a considerable epistemic constraint on prognostic certainty. That problem also exists in subacute and chronic care settings, where decisions about rehabilitation services and the living environment can have an impact on the potential for future recovery (Willems et al. 2015). The interaction between diagnosis and prognosis is important here. Diagnosis of chronic DoC predicts a grim prognosis. Prognosis can prompt clinical pessimism and the forgoing of neurorehabilitation, resulting in self-reinforcing or self-fulfilling prophecies. The snake bites its own tail and the vicious circle closes when the perception of diagnostic and prognostic determinism leads to persistent misdiagnosis (as in Terry Wallis's situation), which in turn reinforces misprognosis (Johnson 2017b; Johnson and Lazaridis 2018).

3.5 Think Globally, Act Locally

DoCs are meant to describe impairments of what we might call "global" states of consciousness, or the overall state of consciousness. Persons in a coma, or under light sedation, or in REM sleep are in different global states of consciousness. Presumably, VS/UWS and MCS patients are also in different global states of consciousness, although the difference is sometimes confusingly called a difference in the "level" of consciousness. It's not clear that a global state of consciousness admits of levels or degrees—it may instead make more sense and be more accurate to think of it as an on/off binary phenomenon. Brain death and coma would be consciousness in the "off" position, while in other DoCs it would be in the "on" position. It's quite plausible that there would be definite experiential differences between being fully aware and being in the MCS, but those differences may have more to do with access to the *contents* of consciousness, what Bayne, Howhy, and Owen (2016) called "local states of consciousness." In ordinary, waking awareness, the contents of consciousness are

> typically available to guide a wide range of cognitive and behavioural processes, such as those involved in verbal report, intentional agency, attentional control, reasoning, executive processing, memory consolidation, and so on. This facet of consciousness is often captured by saying that the contents of consciousness are globally available for the control of thought and action. (2016)[6]

In a state of diminished awareness, such as sedation, the contents may not be fully accessible—sedated patients can sometimes perceive low-level features of objects like color and motion but are unable to categorize a round shape as a ball or to entertain complex thoughts about the rolling red ball. That is, while global consciousness might be binary, phenomenal or local states of consciousness might not be, admitting of multiple possible combinations and degrees of intensity of awareness, including phenomenal states not accessible in a way that can guide or prompt action and behaviors (such as the behaviors key to diagnosing DoCs). Although diagnosis of DoCs is intended to capture and differentiate global states (or levels) of consciousness, it does so by looking for the presence

---

[6] Note here the similarity to Block's access consciousness (A-consciousness), as distinct from phenomenal consciousness (P-consciousness), which refers more explicitly to the contents of consciousness.

of local states, or nonreflexive behavioral proxies for awareness and phenomenal states. It looks for the contents of consciousness, *consciousness of something*. The CRS-R, for example, looks at numerous behaviors that would indicate perception and cognition, such as visual pursuit, fixation, and startle; object localization (e.g., reaching for an object); the ability to follow verbal commands (e.g., "Look up" or "Touch your nose"); verbal and nonverbal communication, and so on. While the ability to follow commands and verbally respond seems clearly to indicate cognition and consciousness of something, it is not necessarily the case that it picks out a "level" of consciousness, nor does the absence of local consciousness, consciousness of something, reliably indicate the absence of global consciousness. Moreover, the absence of behavioral proxies for local states of consciousness can be explained in a number of ways (for example, by sensory impairments, aphasia, and apraxia) that are compatible with consciousness in the global sense. In principle, there is no reason to think that the contents of consciousness must be globally available, or that global consciousness is diminished by the loss of some (or perhaps all) of the local, phenomenal contents of consciousness. Persons without some local sensory percepts—for example, those with inherited deafness—are nonetheless conscious in the global sense, and their consciousness also has local, phenomenal content.

Cognitively intact, typical adult humans can self-report concerning their consciousness and conscious states. This is not a reliable way of distinguishing between those atypical, cognitively compromised humans who are conscious and those who are unconscious. Behaviors like command-following are proxies for mental capacities, but the inability to reliably manifest behaviors that indicate the presence of the capacity being evaluated is one reason someone might "fail" a test of consciousness. The detection of covert brain responses using active neuroimaging paradigms (fMRI, EEG) can sometimes skirt this problem. Patients diagnosed in a VS/UWS have been able to follow commands by controlling their brain activity

(Monti et al. 2010), and they have demonstrated awareness by following the plot of a Hitchcock movie, as evidenced by displaying "highly synchronized brain activity in supramodal frontal and parietal regions, which support executive function" (Naci et al. 2014). These kinds of assessments detect neural proxies of high-level cognition. There is no reason to think that every conscious individual must be able to execute any or all of these covert behaviors given the heterogeneity of brains, brain development, brain injuries, and encephalopathies. Consciousness might still be "on" in those who are not capable of following commands or following the plot of a thriller. Infants can do neither, and dogs are surely conscious even if they are unable to follow the plot of a movie. But dogs have capacities and conscious contents—like their enhanced ability to smell—such that the richness and variety of their olfactory percepts and their olfactory cognition are not available to typical humans (Gadbois and Reeve 2014). That is, there are thoughts dogs can think because of the things they can smell. Young children have less sensory integration than adults, and are able to keep distinct phenomenal information separate, enhancing their ability to discriminate, and to "outperform adults when discriminating stimuli in which these information sources conflict" (Nardini, Bedford, and Mareschal 2010). The point is, there is unknown variety in the percepts, in the phenomenal character of experiences, and in cognitive contents and capacities across humans and across species, but they give us "no reason to suppose that the global states of consciousness had by infants and non-human animals when they are alert and awake are distinct from those had by neurotypical adult humans" (Bayne, Hohwy, and Owen 2016), and likewise for humans with symptoms of impaired consciousness.

The upshot is that behavioral proxies used to identify global states of consciousness—like DoCs—are ill suited to the task, and indeed may be confusing or conflating global and local states of consciousness. The absence of the latter does not indicate the absence of the former. It's not even obvious that the absence of all local states, of all phenomenal awareness, entails a loss of global consciousness. We might well ask what one would be *conscious of* if cut off from all sensory percepts. Perhaps one would be aware of one's own thinking, like Descartes, or perhaps one would be aware of nothing, a sort of idling state, like the wakefulness without awareness hypothesized in VS/UWS patients. Laura Specker-Sullivan, borrowing from Japanese Buddhist thought, has suggested that something like "pure awareness" might be possible in DoCs. She described pure experience, a kind of intrinsic activity of the brain, as

> immediate, without any cognition, deliberation, or judgment; it is the direct experience of a color or sound, without thinking "this is red" or "this sounds pleasant to me" . . . a level of consciousness that precedes the differentiation of subject and object; it is an objectless experience, but it is also a subjectless experience. (2018, 111)

Pure experience is consciousness without awareness of self or the external environment; essentially, exactly the opposite of the kind of consciousness clinical tests look for. Necessarily, this kind of intransitive consciousness—consciousness as a state of being—is clinically untestable, and as Specker-Sullivan has pointed out, it can only be inferred from transitive consciousness (consciousness *of something*).

This mirrors the current state of affairs when it comes to DoCs—the need to infer global from local consciousness. We might well ask—we *should* ask if we think consciousness is morally relevant—about the moral significance and value of any of these types of consciousness, and whether the kind of consciousness we care about can be tested, detected, or verified reliably, or at all. In the next part of the book, I consider those questions, and the question that follows from them: Given epistemic constraints on our ability to reliably identify and verify states of consciousness, what ethical weight can and should consciousness bear?

PART II

THE ETHICS
OF UNCERTAINTY

4

Inference and Inductive Risk

There are several types of inferences common in the diagnosis of brain injury and in prognosis after brain injury. These inferences, although necessary, introduce uncertainty into diagnosis and prognosis. In this chapter, I discuss these different types of inferences and the idea of *inductive risk*, which suggests limits on tolerable ethical risks in the context of medical uncertainty. The uncertainty is ineliminable, but it might be possible to limit its most worrisome impacts.

4.1 Inferences

Different types of inferences are used at various decision points in the aftermath of brain injuries. They are used because there can be no direct access or confirmation of another's conscious states in the absence of a reporting subject. These inferences introduce uncertainty into diagnosis and prognosis.

Abductive inferences are inferences to the best explanation. Abductive inference is the primary inference made in the bedside behavioral diagnosis of disorders of consciousness (DoCs). It goes like this: People who are conscious have reflexive and nonreflexive behavioral responses to stimuli. Importantly, typically functioning conscious adults have nonreflexive responses. They can follow commands. They can verbally respond to questions. From their responsiveness, we can infer that they are conscious. They behave as if they are conscious, and moreover, they behave in ways we think would not be possible if they were not conscious. There are, of course, limits to this inference. In atypical humans—for example, those with sensory or cognitive impairments—responsiveness might also be atypical. Conscious nonhumans will not respond in the same ways that typical humans do. Nonetheless, the basis of the behavioral bedside exam is the inference that someone who does not have nonreflexive behavioral responses to stimuli is not conscious. In other words, the best explanation for someone not *behaving* as if they are conscious is that they are not conscious. An obvious epistemic limit on the abductive inference is that it is most informative with typically functioning adult humans, but humans with DoCs are not typically functioning. Impaired or absent consciousness is but one possible explanation for that.

Reverse inferences also have a role in the context of DoCs, because they are used in the active neuroimaging paradigms that can sometimes uncover covert consciousness in individuals who are behaviorally unresponsive (Poldrack 2011). There are two inferences made. The first one is abductive and involves using neuroimaging to observe brain activity in a healthy (typically functioning, conscious) control subject. The subject is asked to perform a mental task that requires consciousness, for example, *imagine you are playing a game of tennis*. Functional magnetic resonance imaging (fMRI) is used to observe what areas of the brain appear to be active. So, the first inference is abductive: the region of the brain that appears active on fMRI is the one being used to perform that task. There are other abductive inferences running in the background. fMRI detects a blood-oxygen-level-dependent (BOLD) signal. It detects localized changes in brain blood flow and blood oxygenation, rather than neural or mental activity. It doesn't read minds. The BOLD signal is a proxy for localized brain activity that correlates with specific mental activities. The inference is that the recruitment of blood and oxygen to the target area indicates activity in that area.

The second, *reverse* inference runs the other way, and occurs when you ask a behaviorally nonresponsive patient with a brain injury to perform the same task. If the same areas of the brain appear to be active, then you infer that they are performing the same mental task, and, therefore, they are conscious (Johnson 2016; Owen et al. 2006). We can make some further inferences from a subject successfully performing a mental task, including that the subject is capable of sensing and understanding commands, that the target areas of their brain function, and that they are able to willfully modulate their brain activity (Monti et al. 2010). Any one of those might be beyond the capabilities of a specific individual (for example, because of localized injury to the brain) and yet that individual may still be conscious. Decades ago, some clinicians observed that a significant number of patients who were misdiagnosed as unconscious had sensory deficits as a result of their brain injuries. Their behavioral unresponsiveness could be explained by those sensory deficits rather than unconsciousness (Andrews et al. 1996). The same impairments can stymie inferential diagnosis with neuroimaging as well.

Inductive inferences are ampliative, meaning the conclusion goes beyond the known evidence. For that reason, they are also contingent—the conclusion might be false, even if all the evidential premises are true. These are common inferences in prognosis following brain injury.

A simple example of an inductive inference is this:

Premise: The sun has risen every day in recorded human history. (*true*)
Premise: The sun rose today. (*true*)
Conclusion: The sun will rise tomorrow. (*probable, but not certain*)

Note that the conclusion goes beyond the premises. The premises are true concerning events that have already happened. The conclusion makes an inference about a future event based on evidence of past events. But the fact that the sun has always risen (so far as we know) doesn't make it necessary that the sun will rise tomorrow. David Hume described this as the problem of induction. We engage in inductive reasoning constantly, attributing causation to events that occur in sequence. Previous sunrises don't *cause* future sunrises, so the conclusion of the inductive inference can't be certain. It can only be probable. For certainty, and to explain causation, we would need some intermediary principle or law that links past observations to future events. The catch is that we can't use inductive reasoning to arrive at such a principle or law. Hume's skeptical solution to the problem of induction was psychological—we just do engage in inductive, causal inferences about our observations. It is how our minds work. Inductive inferences can be used to prognosticate about future astronomical events, but are also common in medical prognosticating, including prognosticating about survival and recovery after brain injury. A confound that thwarts prognostic inductive inferences is the self-fulfilling prophecy—when prognostication prompts actions that guarantee that the prognosis will come true.

4.2 Prognostic Inferences and Brain Injury

4.2.1 Acute Brain Injuries and Coma

Prognosis in acute brain injuries involves an inductive inference that employs various types of evidence about an injury and a patient. The evidence includes the etiology and severity of the brain injury and information about the patient, such as their age and general health status. The prognosis for recovery is better and more likely following traumatic brain injuries compared to anoxic/hypoxic brain injuries, but the severity of injury matters as well. Some types of brain injury, such as strokes, are more common among older patients, and their outcomes tend to be worse for all the reasons that older patients generally do worse than younger patients. Because inductive inferences are ampliative and go beyond the evidence, even if the objective, observable, empirical evidence is certain, the prognostic inference cannot be certain.

Decisions about treatment and treatment withdrawal must be made for, and about, specific, individual patients. This can involve inductive inferences from past patients, and the use of statistical data from past patients. There are prognostic models and statistical evidence for acute brain injuries, such as the Glasgow Outcome Scale, but nothing currently exists with a sufficiently high level of sensitivity and specificity at the level of individual patients to enable certainty concerning prognostic predictions (Geurts et al. 2014). Among other shortcomings, the mode of death, such as death following withdrawal of life-sustaining treatment (LST), is frequently not explicitly reported in patient data, and patients are rarely followed long term, over years, so outcome measures are frequently limited to time of hospital discharge and 6 months after discharge. That temporal window doesn't reflect the time course of recovery for many patients, for whom "improvements may take significantly longer to manifest" (Lazaridis 2019).

Physicians have their own experiences with patients to draw on in prognosticating about the probable outcome for an individual patient. Those outcomes include death, survival with physical and/or cognitive disability, survival with a DoC, or survival with complete recovery. As with other inductive inferences, the prognosis about an individual patient is contingent, and it may turn out to be incorrect. Prognosis in neurointensive care is also susceptible to covert value judgments about the future quality of life of the patient. Physicians tend to be pessimistic and underestimate good outcomes, overestimate poor outcomes, and seriously underestimate quality of life, and these attitudes and biases may influence their predictions about outcomes for individual patients (Rabinstein and Hemphill 2010; Rocker et al. 2004; Kaufmann et al. 1992). In part this is a product of inductive inferences. Neurointensivists see patients with severe and devastating brain injuries in the days and weeks after injury, when some will die and others will leave the hospital without recovering consciousness, or with severe disability.

Despite the uncertainty, predictions about patient outcomes are commonly made in the period shortly after acute brain injury, when the withdrawal of LST is highly likely to result in death. The prognosis for survival or recovery with continued care is at that point quite uncertain (Wilkinson 2011; Kitzinger and Kitzinger 2013). There is a perceived risk that the patient will recover sufficiently to be independent of LST, but will survive with a disability that will not be acceptable to the patient. That patient will, in Thomas Cochrane's words, be "stuck with life" (Cochrane 2009). Consider the New Jersey Supreme Court's view of the "unendurable" life Karen Ann Quinlan was forced to endure. Or the UK High Court's view that Tony Bland's spirit had already left him, leaving only "a shell of a body." Avoiding the worst outcome for the patient— survival when death would be preferable—comes at a cost: forgoing any possibility of survival with an acceptable outcome (Kitzinger and Kitzinger 2013).

4.2.2 Disorders of Consciousness

Because DoC patients, if they survive to discharge from the hospital, move to nursing facilities or family homes, long-term outcomes are rarely documented, and this influences prognosis and encourages pessimism in acute care, where medical staff are more likely to witness patient deaths or patients who leave neurointensive care while still unconscious. Terry Wallis lived in a nursing home after leaving the hospital, and although his early recovery was observed by his family, recovering the ability to speak took 19 years. Had that not happened, it is unlikely his recovery of consciousness would have been medically documented. There is no way to know how many Terry Wallises there are out there. Studies that have followed patients for several years found that a significant number—about 20 percent—had good recoveries, including return to school and work, 5 years after hospitalization. Others recovered consciousness long after they were considered "permanently" unconscious, calling into question the accepted temporal boundaries for recovery of consciousness, as well as the prognostic accuracy of negative predictors—that is, predictors of poor outcomes (Steppacher, Kaps, and Kissler 2014, 2016).

> UWS [unresponsive wakefulness syndrome] and MCS [minimally conscious state] do not become permanent after 1 year. There are patients with various etiologies recovering after several years in stable UWS or MCS. Finally, the care setting was related to the likelihood of recovery and with appropriate therapy even more patients might regain consciousness after being in UWS and MCS for several years. Thus, patients should have access to reexamination and optimal care including rehabilitative therapies even if the success of these therapies cannot be seen immediately. (2014)

As discussed in the previous chapter, there has been a decades-long problem of misdiagnosis in DoCs (Andrews et al. 1996; van Erp et al. 2015, 2019). The problem persists because diagnosis is behavioral and inferential, an abductive inference. The misdiagnoses are false negatives—patients are diagnosed as unconscious, in a vegetative state/unresponsive wakefulness syndrome (VS/UWS)—when they are in fact conscious. They might be in a MCS, or they might be more than minimally conscious. There is lingering uncertainty about whether "late" recoveries are actually exceptional, unexpected recoveries, or whether extended recoveries are not unusual. It further complicates the misdiagnosis picture that patients can change over time, so that even if they were correctly diagnosed initially, they may recover consciousness covertly, or in a setting like a nursing home where subtle signs of awareness might be misinterpreted or undetected.

Misdiagnosis and misprognosis matter morally. When patients are aware and sentient, they may experience pain or distress that is neglected if they are thought to be unconscious. In terms of decision-making for these patients, in the United States the legal environment is quite different for MCS patients than it is for VS/UWS patients. There is long-standing precedent for surrogates to withdraw LST when patients are in the VS/UWS, going back to the *Quinlan* case in 1976. The courts have rejected withdrawing artificial nutrition and hydration (ANH) from MCS patients several times, or they have maintained near-impossible standards for evidence of patient wishes, and, although every state has included the vegetative state or unconsciousness as a triggering condition for withholding or withdrawing LST, no states have yet included the MCS or cognitive motor dissociation (CMD; Johnson and Cerminara 2020).[1]

4.2.3 Inferences about Quality of Life

The last set of inferences are the ones made about quality of life. Quality of life is individual and subjective. The person experiencing a life can know about its subjective quality, but the outside observer

---

[1] In a 2020 case in Florida, *In re: Guardianship of Lizbeth Young*, the trial court held that there was clear and convincing evidence that ending life-prolonging treatment for the patient, Lizbeth Young, was in her best interests. Young was a 64-year-old woman with a history of childhood brain injury and chronic mental illness. Her guardian petitioned the court for authorization to consent to end LST. Young was in the MCS, and had no known previously expressed preferences regarding treatment. Her feeding tube caused harmful side effects, such as infections, fluid accumulation "so bad that it seeped through the pores of her skin," low blood pressure, gastrointestinal bleeding, and skin ulcers. Young had advanced dementia, a terminal condition. It was unknown if she could feel pain. One of her doctors told the court that continuing treatment was "almost cruel" (*In re: Young* 2020). Young's fragile health and terminal illness make the court's decision about her best interests not straightforwardly about the MCS, and it is unlikely to set a new precedent for withdrawing LST from MCS patients.

can have only a very sketchy understanding of it. We might observe behavioral or physiological evidence of pain or distress, or pleasure, but without a first-person report, the picture is incomplete. (A very good actor, for example, could convince us that they are suffering deeply and existentially, or that they are experiencing the heights of joy, and convince us of something about their quality of life, but it would be an illusion.) We don't know much about what life is like with impaired consciousness, because affected individuals cannot meaningfully communicate.

There has been extensive research on quality of life among disabled persons, however. The majority of disabled people, including locked-in patients, consistently report that their own quality of life is good (Lulé et al. 2009; Bruno et al. 2011). This contrasts with the perceptions and beliefs held by non-disabled people (including caregivers) about the quality of life of those with disabilities. This mismatch between common perceptions and the quality of life reported by disabled persons is called the disability paradox. The paradox is a misnomer—it implies that there is something absurd or contradictory about having good quality of life with disability. Explanations for the lack of congruence between disabled persons and others tend to focus on the disabled person as the locus of the mismatch. One response is to assume that disabled persons lack self-awareness and are unreliable reporters of their own quality of life. This view should be dismissed. It is grounded in epistemic, testimonial injustice, in which the reliability of an individual's knowledge and testimony are discounted, due to prejudice, in favor of other knowers and speakers (Fricker 2007). It's important to recognize how the disability paradox is paradoxical only because of implicit and explicit biases that valorize being able-bodied.

Another explanation is the phenomenon of "response shift," a recalibration or reprioritization of value in persons living with disabilities, such that they assess pain or impairments differently, or modify the relative importance of different domains of life (Dijkers 2004; Johnson 2013; Schwartz et al. 2007). Attributing the subjective experience of positive quality of life to response shift is another instance of epistemic and testimonial injustice. It assumes that there is some objective standard—life without disability—and that disabled individuals have effectively downgraded their expectations in response to disability: They've settled for less, but, more importantly, they have a false or mistaken belief that it is not less. A safer assumption, one not informed by ableist bias or epistemic injustice, is that disabled persons, like everyone else, must adjust to changes in their lives and circumstances. When those changes involve acquired disabilities, they can be highly disruptive, affecting many aspects of life, including a person's self-identity. But other significant changes in life—the loss of a job, a change in career, a natural disaster, having a child—can also be highly disruptive and require adjustment.

The real paradox is why there is a persistent belief that quality of life is poor for disabled persons despite evidence to the contrary. If able-bodied persons have the epistemic authority to judge their own quality of life, so, too, should disabled persons. This includes disabled persons with brain injuries and cognitive and communication differences who can still be authorities regarding their own quality of life.

The inferences made about quality of life are value judgments about the quality and value of life for disabled persons—some would say they also place a value *on* the lives of disabled persons. At best, these are inferences by analogy, where the analogy is to what non-disabled individuals—or doctors—consider a good, worthwhile life. We should be worried not only that prognosis in neurointensive care is inferential and uncertain, but also that it is very susceptible to covert—or overt—value judgments about the quality of life of persons with brain injuries and disabilities.

4.3 Self-fulfilling Prophecies as an Epistemic Confound

It is clear that DoCs are among the most feared and worst perceived outcomes physicians and families seek to avoid by withdrawing LST. It is frequently presumed that quality of life will be poor, and it is in the patient's interests, or aligns with the patient's values and preferences, to avoid a chronic DoC. Thus, there is considerable entanglement of the inferences made in neurointensive care and inferences about DoCs. Because of the time pressure to withdraw treatment while patients remain comatose and dependent on a ventilator, many decisions to withdraw treatment occur within the first 72 hours following injury (Turgeon et al. 2011), and withdrawal of LST is the leading factor in neurointensive care unit deaths, preceding up to 70 percent of deaths (Turgeon et al. 2011; Côte et al. 2013; Izzy et al. 2013; Verkade et al. 2012). The percentage of deaths that follow withdrawals has increased over time, despite improvements in neurointensive care. To say the deaths were "caused by" withdrawal of LST only means that withdrawal of LST was the proximate cause of death. It does not imply that all of those patients would have survived if treatment had continued. Indeed, some would have died regardless, although some would have survived.

A prognosis of death becomes a self-fulfilling prophecy when a significant number of deaths occur because the prognosis prompts withdrawal of LST. That reinforces the inference that patients with severe brain injuries will die. Indeed, the prognosis of death all but guarantees that some patients will die, not because the prognosis itself is certain, but because it precipitates actions with a certain outcome—death. And virtually all die if LST is withdrawn. Of course, some patients will die even if LST is continued. Of those who survive to hospital discharge, some will also die later (Anke et al. 2015; Steppacher, Kaps, and Kissler 2014). Self-fulfilling prophecies create a serious epistemic challenge to the validity and strength of prognostic inferences. They skew the evidence. There might be high mortality among patients with brain injuries, but it might also be that high levels of mortality are caused by predictions of mortality and unacceptable outcomes that prompt withdrawal of LST. It cannot be known if they are accurate prophecies, or merely self-fulfilling. Even more troubling are the ethical implications. People who might have survived to have good and flourishing lives will die avoidable deaths. Self-fulfilling prophecies increase the risks of being wrong.

4.4 Inductive Risk

Inductive risk is a concept that was introduced in philosophy of science the 1950s. It explains two interacting risks of accepting a scientific hypothesis—epistemic and ethical risks—and it connects epistemic and ethical duties. In its classic formulation, it demonstrates that ethical judgments have an important and expansive role to play in science, a simple (but not uncontroversial) idea. Richard Rudner put it this way: how great a risk you should be willing to take in being wrong will depend on how ethically serious the consequences are if you make a mistake (Rudner 1953). As Heather Douglas put it, non-epistemic values must guide decision-making in science in situations where there is inductive risk (Douglas 2000). The basic idea is that science does not operate in an ethical vacuum, free of non-epistemic, ethical constraints. This should be a no-brainer.

One kind of inductive risk is epistemic risk. That is just the risk of getting the wrong answer or accepting an incorrect hypothesis. There are also non-epistemic risks, which we can just call ethical risks, or the ethically significant consequences of being wrong. Just as inductive inferences cannot be certain, inductive reasoning cannot prove beyond doubt any hypothesis. The problem of inductive risk is this: given uncertainty, what is the appropriate epistemic standard of evidence for accepting a hypothesis? Rudner's classic formulation proposes that the tolerable level of epistemic risk or uncertainty varies, and it should be limited by the ethical risks of being wrong. That is, ethically significant consequences of being wrong should constrain epistemic decisions about accepting a hypothesis. This is the *Principle of Inductive Risk*. In §4.4.3, I introduce a novel second principle, so this one will be called the First Principle of Inductive Risk.

4.4.1 The First Principle of Inductive Risk

Rudner uses an example comparing the manufacturing of belt buckles and pharmaceuticals. A defective (garment) belt buckle might cause someone's pants to fall down, which is not that serious as ethical risks go. So, we can tolerate a lot of uncertainty concerning reliability and efficacy when it comes to belt buckles. Manufacturing pharmaceuticals, on the other hand, involves a lot of ethically significant risks, like death, illness, injury, or permanent disability. The First Principle of Inductive Risk tells us that our epistemic standard—our level of certainty about safety and efficacy—should be quite high when it comes to pharmaceutical manufacturing, because the ethical risks are quite high.

The First Principle of Inductive Risk is useful in bioethics and in medicine. Consider again prenatal screening. Prenatal screening of fetuses can detect Trisomy 21 (T21), which involves a spectrum and range of disability. Importantly, the type or severity of disability cannot be detected or predicted prenatally. Pregnancy terminations are common after a prenatal diagnosis of T21. Prenatal tests can also involve some risk to a pregnancy, including the risk of miscarriage and the loss of a wanted pregnancy, and there are risks of false negatives, where the tests fail to detect anomalies, and a small risk of false positives.[2] Prenatal testing can also detect fetal anomalies that are considered incompatible with life, so-called lethal malformations where fetal or neonatal death is likely. Anencephaly, in which the brain does not develop, is considered lethal, and neonatal survival is frequently measured in hours. Yet there are cases of survival beyond the newborn period for this and many other conditions considered lethal, and so concerns about self-fulfilling prophecies arise—if a neonate has a condition judged to be incompatible with life, life-saving treatments, including resuscitation, may not be attempted (Wilkinson et al. 2012). Thus, there are some epistemic risks with prenatal screening—risks of false positives or false negatives, and risks that involve the inability to accurately predict outcomes. But there are also non-epistemic risks, because decisions are made on the basis of prenatal tests, decisions that affect who is born.

We can apply the First Principle of Inductive Risk to evaluations of the level of epistemic risk involved in prenatal screening, which includes a number of epistemic uncertainties. The tolerable level of epistemic risk will vary with the ethical risks, and the ethical risks are not fixed or universal, given variation in the physical and psychological effects for pregnant persons; the moral, religious, and cultural status of the fetus; individual values; and individual and social variation in acceptance of disability and access to resources for disabled persons. Thus, unlike the case of manufacturing belt buckles, where we have risks that are relatively minor, easily characterized, and invariable, the risks involved in prenatal screening are highly variable, including at the level of individual values and risk-aversion, and they include some very serious risks: the loss of a wanted pregnancy and the preventable birth (and

---

[2] Emily Rapp wrote movingly of her son Ronan's brief life in *The Still Point of the Turning World*. Ronan had Tay-Sachs disease, a progressive, inevitably fatal disorder that affects young children beginning in infancy. Rapp was herself born with a congenital limb difference, and although while pregnant with Ronan she had prenatal testing for Tay-Sachs, the results produced a false negative (Rapp 2014).

death) of a child with a fatal disorder. The seriousness of the ethical risks calls for a correspondingly low level of tolerable epistemic risk. Put another way, given the serious ethical risks, and the kinds of ethical decisions prenatal screening provokes, the First Principle of Inductive Risk tells us that prenatal screening demands a high level of diagnostic and prognostic certainty.

What does the First Principle of Inductive Risk look like when applied to decision-making concerning brain injuries? There exists a variable level of prognostic uncertainty about the patient's future should they survive a brain injury. There is a high level of ethical risk in withdrawing LST—near certainty that the patient will die, and also some unknown but serious risk that the patient will lose an opportunity to survive with a good, flourishing life. Correspondingly, our epistemic standards should be quite high, or, put another way, a low level of epistemic, prognostic uncertainty is tolerable given the serious ethical risks of being wrong.

4.4.2 False Negatives and False Positives

There is a high risk of false negatives in bedside behavioral exams of DoC patients—considerable risk that a patient is diagnosed as unconscious when they are minimally, or more than minimally, conscious. Thus, the choice of methodology for diagnosing DoCs also involves inductive risk. There is a significant risk—40 percent—of getting a false negative. A false positive would mean an unconscious patient is misdiagnosed as conscious. Douglas has argued that in setting standards for statistical significance, "one must decide what balance between false positives and false negatives is optimal. In making this decision, one ought to consider the consequences of the false positives and false negatives, both epistemic and non-epistemic" (Douglas 2000, 567). We could and should also choose whether it is better to have false positives or false negatives in the diagnosis of DoCs.

In general, false positives in medicine are undesirable. They can subject patients to unnecessary diagnostic procedures and treatments. A false positive diagnosis of consciousness—the determination that an unconscious patient is conscious—could have undesirable consequences, including treatment when the patient would not have chosen treatment, or continued life when the patient would not have chosen to live, as well as a range of possible emotional, psychological, and financial effects for the patient's family and caregivers. False negatives are also undesirable. A misdiagnosis of unconsciousness in a conscious patient can lead to undertreatment of pain, denial of rehabilitation, withdrawal of treatment, death when the patient would have chosen life, medical and psychosocial neglect, and an inaccurate prognosis of the potential for recovery. We could argue over whether a false negative or a false positive is worse in the context of DoCs. Both are worse than an accurate diagnosis, but from a patient-centered view, the false negative has the potential to be far worse for the patient who experiences undertreated or untreated pain, discomfort, and distress, and who is psychosocially neglected and understimulated. The unconscious patient who is treated as if they were conscious will not suffer physically or psychologically, but the fulfillment of their preferences concerning treatment and LST may be thwarted. The non-epistemic badness of a false positive or false negative will be, to some extent, subjective and individual, but it will also have familial, social, and societal repercussions.

Ideally, we want neither false positives nor false negatives. In practice, we must choose the right balance of the two. We currently have a high rate of false negatives in diagnoses of DoCs. Let's simplify things a bit and identify overtreatment and undertreatment as the consequences of false positives and false negatives, respectively. They are risks that are general across medical diagnosis. Obviously, there are other consequences when it comes to DoCs, including avoidable deaths and undesired lives, but for the sake of simplicity, let's set those aside for now. Balancing false negatives and positives requires that we choose to go one way or the other, and so we must weigh the non-epistemic consequences: overtreatment and undertreatment (this assumes, of course, that overtreatment is possible, which it is not in places that are medically underresourced).

At present, there is no gold standard diagnostic test for DoCs, because the most widely used, clinically accepted tests do not meet the criteria for accuracy to be considered "gold" standard. But they are standard. They are also unacceptably vulnerable to false negatives. By almost any measure, a 40 percent error rate is unacceptably high, but the problem is exacerbated when the ethical risks include neglect, undertreatment, and unwanted death. Ideally, we want tests that are less prone to epistemic error when being wrong has significant ethical risks. In our non-ideal clinical world, an alternative is to reduce non-epistemic, ethically important errors by indexing our ethical risk-taking to the epistemic risks of being wrong.

4.4.3 The Second Principle of Inductive Risk

The concept of inductive risk is useful if we flip it and constrain ethical risk-taking in the presence of epistemic uncertainty. That is what the Second Principle of Inductive Risk does.

The Second Principle of Inductive Risk tells us that the acceptable level of ethical risk varies and should be constrained by the level of epistemic (scientific, medical) uncertainty.

By ethical risks I still mean ethically relevant risks, such as death, injury, and illness. But the second principle applies in circumstances where our non-epistemic decisions are specifically ethically fraught, such as decisions to continue or discontinue LST or to limit or withhold treatment. And the level of acceptable risk-taking in making those decisions would be set by the level of medical uncertainty about diagnosis or prognosis. In acute brain injury and coma, where there is often a great deal of medical uncertainty, a low level of ethical risk-taking would be tolerable. That would seem to rule out withdrawal of LST in the first few days after injury, when uncertainty is heightened. With other DoCs, there is also a lot of epistemic uncertainty. Four in ten patients are misdiagnosed. So, a low level of ethical risk-taking is tolerable. According to the second principle, then, there will be circumstances in which decisions to withdraw LST would be judged intolerably risky.

The Second Principle of Inductive Risk does not have set thresholds for acceptable ethical risks. It requires us to set a threshold that corresponds appropriately to the level of medical uncertainty that exists. When we do this, we can take into consideration factors like formal or informal advance decision-making by the patient and the patient's own values and tolerance for risk. Indeed, there will be circumstances where the level of epistemic risk is high, but other factors, including individual preferences, will set the bar low for ethical risk-taking.

To summarize: The First Principle of Inductive Risk tells us to index epistemic risk-taking to the ethical risks of being wrong. The greater the ethical risks of being wrong, the less epistemic risk we should tolerate. The Second Principle of Inductive Risk tells us to index ethical risk-taking to the epistemic risks of being wrong. There, the greater the epistemic risk (of being wrong), the less tolerance we should have for ethical risk-taking. The two principles are subtly different, in that they constrain different types of risks—epistemic and ethical.

The second principle cautions us against early withdrawals of LST and other treatments, both because the level of uncertainty soon after brain injury is high, and because that uncertainty—and the corresponding risks—are further heightened by withdrawals that lead to death and self-fulfilling prophecies. That is, the ethical risks are heightened by epistemic uncertainty, and ought to be constrained by that uncertainty. But the epistemic risks are in turn heightened by ethically risky choices that result in self-fulfilling prophecies.

5

Upstream/Downstream

In contemplating whether to withdraw life-sustaining treatment (LST) shortly after serious brain injuries, surrogates weigh the risks and benefits of future life. The risks include very short-term risks when the prognosis for survival is bleak. Similarly, when individuals make those decisions for themselves in advance directives, or through anticipatory discussions with their healthcare providers and proxies, they may be imagining a future that is in some subjectively important sense undesirable, and they may decide against it. Those decisions can be deeply personal, based on individual values and goals and on prior experience, including experiences with the illness and death of loved ones. Those decisions can also be misinformed or overly pessimistic. Some people believe that life with a brain injury or disability is inevitably a deficient, undesirable life of poor quality and diminished opportunities, and they choose not to risk such a life. Some surrogates believe that the patient they are deciding for would not want to live a life they would judge to be missing the experiences and capacities they believe are necessary for a good and flourishing life.

I am less worried about the choices made by individuals deciding for themselves. The advance choices made by autonomous individuals about future possibilities are rarely fully informed—how can they be? But whether we think they are mistaken or not, they ought to be respected for independent reasons. We can presumptively grant that a person's self-knowledge is adequate and has sufficient epistemic authority. People have the right to act on their individual values and preferences, however quirky or unconventional or imperfect, when it comes to their own bodies, lives, and deaths.[1]

My concern is with the decisions made by surrogates and medical staff, and with risk inversion. Risk inversion occurs when greater, certain, immediate risks are undertaken to prevent lesser or merely speculative future risks. There is risk inversion in what I call upstream and downstream risks in the context of brain injury and disorders of consciousness (DoCs), where more certain risks are undertaken upstream (in neurointensive care) to avoid less certain, more speculative risks downstream, later. In particular, I'm concerned with ethical risks—or risks that have ethically important consequences. As discussed in previous chapters, there is a great deal of uncertainty concerning prognosis after brain injuries, and that uncertainty increases the ethical riskiness of some actions.

The upstream action in this context is withdrawing LST from comatose patients with brain injuries in neurointensive care. This involves significant risk. The action is intended to result in the death of the patient, with one of two goals: (1) to prevent a prolonged death in case the patient is expected to die no matter what is done, or (2) to prevent the uncertain downstream risk that the patient will survive with a life that is undesirable. In the worst case, the patient may survive but wish they had not. My focus here is on the second scenario.

Consider a nonmetaphorical upstream/downstream scenario, where polluted water from a manufacturing facility is dumped into a river upstream of a village that depends on the water for agriculture. When the polluted water travels downstream, it will cause harm to the villagers. Preventing harm to the villagers requires taking action upstream, by preventing the factory from dumping polluted water into the river. Here, the costs and risks to the factory and to the villagers can be anticipated well enough. For the

[1] The usual exceptions apply. We do not have the right to willfully and knowingly endanger others, by spreading infectious diseases, for example.

sake of simplicity, we can suppose that it would cost relatively little to treat the water upstream, and there is no loss of benefit to the villagers in doing so. Taking action upstream to prevent greater harm downstream makes sense, and indeed there is an ethical imperative to do it.

This may be the kind of upstream calculation being made in decisions to withdraw LST. The greater harm, the one to be avoided, would be living life in an undesirable condition. That "a fate worse than death" is a commonly used phrase populated with innumerable possibilities evinces the extent to which humans view death as one of many possible evils, and not always the greatest evil. So, when I say that near certain death is a greater upstream risk undertaken to prevent the lesser downstream risk of disability, I refer not to the extent to which the risks in question are bad or undesirable—which is importantly subjective and individual—but rather to the level of greater or lesser certainty involved. It may well be that death is the greater or the lesser evil in some cases. We can safely assume here that some proportion of survivors of brain injury will indeed have lives so undesirable that they would prefer they had not lived. For persons looking ahead to possible futures, being chronically unconscious—for years, or perhaps for life—would be such a life. Some of those persons would rather risk losing out on a possibly good life than risk their worst-case scenario. But some other proportion of survivors will have lives of neutral value—neither better nor worse than before. Some will have lives that are slightly worse, but still well worth living. Some will have better lives than before, since the goods (and evils) of life are many and various. Some people survive brain injuries with few or minor impairments and loss of function, some with more disabling impairments or loss of function, and some will make a full recovery and their lives will eventually be much as they were before. The chief source of uncertainty about which of these outcomes will occur is that many decisions to withdraw LST are made in the hours soon after brain injuries, when prognosis is highly uncertain. Limited longitudinal follow-up of patients with brain injuries adds to the uncertainty of prognostication about long-term outcomes. Those upstream decisions, then, result in a risk inversion, where a higher level of risk is undertaken upstream—certain death—to prevent a less certain risk downstream.

5.1 The Window of Opportunity

The so-called window of opportunity is the period shortly after a brain injury when a patient is still ventilator dependent, and when LST can be withdrawn, leading to death in a short period of time. Death is a virtual certainty (Turgeon et al. 2011). Prognosis about future recovery, however, is still very uncertain in many cases (Lazaridis 2019). The window of opportunity creates time pressure to make decisions about withdrawing LST, because the window may close. When it closes, there is a perceived risk that the patient may survive in a condition that they would not have chosen for themselves or would not find acceptable (Wilkinson 2011; Kitzinger and Kitzinger 2013).

Because of the time pressure to act before the window closes, decisions to withdraw LST frequently occur within the first 72 hours after a brain injury. As Turgeon et al. noted,

> The high proportion of deaths in all centres following withdrawal of life-sustaining therapy, specifically in the early phase of care, is concerning when placed in the context of limited ability to accurately determine prognosis for patients with severe traumatic brain injury. (2011, 7)

The window of opportunity contributes to premature and possibly avoidable deaths, but it also throws an epistemic monkey wrench into attempts at evidence-based prognostication by corrupting the evidence for survival. That the number of neurointensive care deaths following withdrawal of LST has increased over the years is evidence of how self-fulfilling prophecies can influence treatment and nontreatment decisions, as well as survival and mortality. The lack of evidence that might confirm or refute pessimistic predictions of death or poor outcomes for patients with brain injuries exacerbates the epistemic uncertainty by creating a false sense of certainty.

The very existence of a so-called window of opportunity for an easier, quicker death upstream implies that such a death is, for at least some, preferable to the downstream alternatives, which are a more protracted and difficult death, or the possibility of chronic disability or chronic DoC.

5.1.1 Slow Closure in DoCs

One reason to wait when the prognosis is a DoC is that recovery occurs on a very different timescale—months to years—than exists in the neurointensive care unit, where time can be measured in hours and days. The vegetative state/unresponsive wakefulness syndrome (VS/UWS) is "persistent" until 3 months after nontraumatic brain injury, and 12 months after traumatic brain injury (TBI). After that, it is considered chronic and stable. A substantial minority of patients *will* recover consciousness beyond these time frames (Giacino et al. 2018). The chances of recovery are not nil. More importantly, patients may still experience functionally significant recovery more than a year post-injury, with some longitudinal studies showing that about 20 percent recover enough to return to work or school (Giacino et al. 2018; Nakase-Richardson et al. 2012). It remains the case that as the period of unresponsiveness endures, recovery of consciousness becomes less likely, and those who recover "late" are more likely to require long-term and supportive care.

There are considerations beyond time that can affect prognosis. Patients who are elderly, extremely premature infants, the medically fragile, or the medically unstable generally have a poorer prognosis for survival, and so immediate decisions regarding the provision of invasive or traumatic treatment, including resuscitation, must often be made. While some decisions, such as Do Not Resuscitate or Do Not Intubate decisions, are time sensitive and may well involve self-fulfilling prophecies, they are less sensitive to the closing of the window of opportunity than treatment and nontreatment decisions made in the acute phase of brain injuries. The mismatch between slow recoveries and quick decisions results in risk inversions.

5.2 Withdrawal of Life-Sustaining Treatment in Neurointensive Care

The haste with which LST is withdrawn in the acute period following brain injuries is sometimes (perhaps often) informed by a belief in "better dead than disabled."

A 1999 study at Columbia University in New York found about 43 percent of deaths among patients with brain injuries followed withdrawal of LST (Mayer and Kossoff 1999). A decade later, a University of Massachusetts study found that withdrawal of care was "the most important predictor of in-hospital mortality" (Izzy et al. 2013, 347), accounting for 68 percent of deaths after brain injury. Among the 232 patients included in the study, 64 percent of patients with severe brain injuries died after withdrawal of LST, and 92 percent of patients with moderate brain injuries died after LST was withdrawn. (The patients with moderate brain injuries were more often elderly, which perhaps explains the seemingly paradoxical greater percentage—when compared to patients with severe brain injuries—of decisions to withdraw LST.) The median intensive care stay for patients who died after treatment was withdrawn was 3 days, less than half the length of stay for other patients, indicating that withdrawal decisions are made within hours of the initial brain injury.

In a Canadian study of six hospitals, 64 percent of brain injury deaths, on average, were associated with withdrawal of LST. There was considerable variability between hospitals, from 30.4 percent to an astounding 92.9 percent (Turgeon et al. 2011; Côte et al. 2013). Many of these deaths (45.6 percent) occurred within the first 3 days of intensive care hospitalization. A 2020 study of withdrawal of LST in severe TBI analyzed 37,949 cases in trauma centers in the United States. LST was withdrawn from 20.74 percent of patients, and 93.7 percent of those died in hospital, with median time to withdrawal of LST being 2 days. By comparison, 18.3 percent of patients who continued treatment died in hospital. In total, 12,987 of the severe TBI patients (33.9 percent) died in hospital, and 54.1 percent of those deaths followed withdrawal of LST. The difference is stark when you compare those who died after withdrawal of LST (93.7 percent) to those who died when treatment was continued (18.3 percent). One can only speculate as to whether any of the patients who died after treatment was withdrawn might have survived, but the numbers do point clearly to the virtual inevitability of death following withdrawal of LST.

The takeaway is that while not everyone dies after a brain injury, the majority of those who die do so after LST is withdrawn. Some of those patients would have died anyway, whether or not LST was withdrawn, but some of them might have survived, and some of them might have had good enough recoveries.

5.3 Withdrawal of Life-Sustaining Treatment and Disorders of Consciousness

Since the *Quinlan* and *Cruzan* decisions, the withdrawal of LST, including ventilators and artificial nutrition and hydration (ANH), from unconscious patients has been widely accepted as permissible under law in the United States and many Western nations, and in ethics. The consensus view that has emerged is that life has no value for someone who is permanently unconscious. Indeed, many people would agree that if they are in a state of permanent unconsciousness, there is little point in being alive. The things we value in life—our families, our friends, our creative endeavors, pastimes, and recreations—would no longer be available to us. This view is not universally shared, of course, and there are individuals, communities, spiritual traditions, and cultures that have a very different view about the value of continued life, and about the morality of withdrawing the means of sustaining life.

At the time of *Quinlan* and *Cruzan*, much that is known today about DoCs was unknown. The VS/UWS was known only as the persistent vegetative state when Karen Ann Quinlan was diagnosed and when the New Jersey Supreme Court ruled that keeping her alive was cruel and unusual. When Nancy Cruzan was diagnosed, and when the Supreme Court decided on her case in 1990, the persistent vegetative state was still the only diagnostic category. It would be 4 more years before temporal boundaries distinguishing the *persistent* from the *permanent* vegetative state would be established and standardized (Multi-Society Task Force on PVS 1994). The Supreme Court has not considered a case involving the minimally conscious state (MCS), but the lower courts in the United States that have done so have consistently ruled against withdrawal of ANH. In the United Kingdom, where courts must grant permission to withdraw LST, they use a "best interests" standard and generally permit withdrawal, although there have been notable exceptions.

Some US states restrict withdrawal of LST from patients lacking decisional capacity, but many carve out an exception for those who are permanently unconscious. New York State's Family Health Care Decisions Act, for example, permits surrogates to withdraw LST if treatment would be extraordinarily burdensome to the patient and the patient can be expected to die within 6 months, or if the patient is permanently unconscious.[2] In several states, surrogates for patients in the MCS have been rebuffed by courts when they attempted to have LST withdrawn (Johnson and Cerminara 2020). Thus, surrogates for patients diagnosed as unconscious may be granted the right to withdraw LST on their behalf, but not surrogates for those in the MCS. Arguably, this establishes a legal double standard that draws a bright, arbitrary line through the liminal boundaries between DoCs, ignoring both diagnostic uncertainties and individual differences and preferences (Johnson 2011).

There are no data available on how frequently LST is withdrawn from chronic DoC patients. While many states have created exceptions for VS/UWS patients, the legal situation complicates decision-making by surrogates in all cases where the patient retains some level of consciousness but did not leave clear and convincing evidence of their preferences regarding treatment.

Thus, another reason to act sooner rather than later after brain injury is that it may be much more legally difficult to withdraw LST later, once the patient has survived the acute injury, and a somewhat clearer prognostic picture is possible. An equally significant consideration is that once the acute phase has passed, the patient may require relatively minimal LST, such as ANH. Many families understandably balk at withdrawing nutrition and hydration, viewing it as death by starvation. This thicket of legal, ethical, and personal considerations creates pressure to make upstream decisions during the acute phase of brain injury, to avoid the risks and the foreclosure of remedies downstream. These considerations encourage risk inversion.

---

[2] New York State Family Health Care Decisions Act (2010). https://www.nysenate. gov/legislation/laws/PBH/2994-D

5.4   Risk Inversion: Downstream Risks and Upstream Risks

In paradigmatic cases of acting upstream to prevent downstream risks, such as polluting waterways, failing to act preventively upstream can have seriously bad consequences downstream, and in some cases, those consequences may not be remediable. If ecosystems are harmed, plants and animals may die. The pollution may be cleaned up through considerable effort and expense, but the death of individual animals is not reversible, nor can we recover a species driven to extinction. Human health may be affected by polluted water as well—perhaps the pollution will cause cancers and people will become severely ill or die.

In the case of brain injuries, when you act upstream, you are creating a risk that exists only because of the attempt to avoid the downstream risk. The risk is missing a chance at possible recovery and life. Acting upstream results in near certain death, whereas the downstream risk is speculative, based on epistemically problematic inferences. That's an inversion of the risks: the upstream strategy with a certain outcome—death—is employed to avoid a merely possible and *possibly bad but also possibly not bad* downstream risk. Since some patients with acute brain injuries will die despite LST, the consequences of inverting the risks are undertaken only by those who might have survived had treatment continued. But it is often very difficult to predict which patients belong to the group who are certain to die even with treatment, and in any case, as noted above, most deaths occur after LST is withdrawn. So minimally, we can say that the risk inversion exists for all (or nearly all) patients for whom withdrawal of LST is considered. When patients are not given the opportunity to survive, self-fulfilling prophecies are inevitable and undermine our ability to prognosticate with any degree of certainty about likely outcomes.

What counts as a good and flourishing life—what is *good for* an individual—is subjective. The capacities I think are necessary for *me* to have a good and flourishing life—to experience well-being in my life—will likely overlap considerably, but not entirely, with what many other people think about their own lives. Devastating brain injuries are not always compatible with life at all and can involve a considerably shortened life. The loss of life, or years of expected life, is a significant loss. The loss of capacities for interaction, for endeavors that are fulfilling, enjoyable, or give one a sense of purpose, and the loss of independence and autonomy, are importantly life-altering, in a negative way, for many adults.

The epistemic and ethical critique of acting hastily to withdraw LST in the aftermath of brain injury in order to avoid disability is that it inverts the risks, accepting death and the risk of missed opportunities to live and live well in order to avoid a less certain risk of living with a disability. An epistemic and ethical critique of the underlying, motivating belief in "better dead than disabled" is that it inverts the risks in a way that leads to decisions that are irrational and inconsistent with reality, or uninformed by known evidence. Catastrophizing disability in this way also contributes to perpetuating the myth that disability is a tragedy that is incompatible with living a good life, and so it also undermines the efforts of existing disabled persons—out there living their good lives—to be accepted and accommodated.

5.5 Futility

The concept of medical futility and futile interventions is ambiguous. One way to think about futility is sometimes referred to as "physiological futility," which describes treatments or interventions that cannot achieve their intended aims. Straightforward examples of this would be attempting to treat a virus using antibiotics or attempting to resuscitate a corpse that has signs of rigor mortis. In both cases, if the aim is to restore health, the intervention cannot succeed.

A more contentious way of thinking about futility looks not at whether certain aims can be achieved through an intervention, but at whether the aim itself is worth pursuing. This is sometimes called "qualitative futility" because what makes the intervention "futile" is that it cannot achieve a qualitatively good aim. An example of this would be attempting to resuscitate an elderly patient with Stage IV lung cancer, where cardiopulmonary resuscitation might succeed, but the patient can be expected to die in the near future. One could question whether the trauma of resuscitation for a patient facing imminent death, and the moral distress of medical staff whose efforts cause that trauma, make it worthwhile to attempt resuscitation, and whether saving that life, if only briefly, is a worthwhile aim. There are, of course, reasons to think it might be. Families might find comfort in knowing that "everything possible" was done for their loved one. The patient might have requested that everything possible be done to extend their life. Refusing a request to attempt resuscitation might result in legal liability, or it might cause the patient's survivors distress.

5.5.1   Mann Ki Lee

In 2010, Mann Ki Lee, a 46-year-old Toronto father with advanced thymic cancer, was admitted to Toronto's Sunnybrook Health Sciences Centre. Lee told doctors he wanted them to use all medical measures possible to save him. He wrote his request in a power of attorney document and confirmed it in a videotaped recording. He was informed of, and understood, the risks of CPR. During his hospitalization, his doctors, in violation of Ontario law, issued a unilateral Do Not Resuscitate (DNR) order, without consulting Lee's family. The doctors, and the hospital, argued that the decision to resuscitate was strictly a medical one, regardless of patient wishes.

Lee's family took the hospital to court, and a judge initially revoked the DNR order. A lawyer for the hospital stated that Lee "should be allowed to die in peace without this gross and monstrous intervention." Lee's brother accused the doctors of "playing God" (Cribb 2010).

Lee's family did eventually agree to the DNR after his condition deteriorated, but they were forced to spend his last days of life in court, fighting his doctors, rather than being by his side.

Personal and familial considerations can rightly override concerns about whether an intervention can achieve a physiological goal, and they highlight the extent to which value judgments and futility judgments are entangled in ways that make the latter ambiguous and not straightforwardly objective.

5.5.2 Potentially Inappropriate Interventions

Efforts to disambiguate the different senses of "futile" and to separate physiological futility from other considerations have had mixed success. There can be a strong case for not attempting interventions that cannot achieve medical aims like prolonging life and restoring health, especially when they can harm patients more than they help. As noted above, however, there can be important psychosocial benefits in attempting them anyway. One effort at separation and disambiguation, in a multi-society policy statement, involves usefully reserving the term *futile* for those interventions that simply cannot achieve intended physiological goals. Where the separation runs into difficulty is in designating as "potentially inappropriate" those medical interventions that could work but that should not be provided for other, "competing ethical considerations" (Bosslet et al. 2015; Kon et al. 2016).

By definition, those "potentially inappropriate" interventions have the potential to achieve intended physiological goals, such as successful resuscitation. They are deemed potentially inappropriate when there is no reasonable expectation that the patient will improve sufficiently to survive outside the acute care setting, or when there is no reasonable expectation that the patient's neurologic function will improve sufficiently to allow the patient to perceive the benefits of treatment. (Kon et al. 2016)

One example of a potentially inappropriate intervention, according to the policy statement, is this: "A clinician believes it is inappropriate to initiate dialysis in a patient in a persistent vegetative state" (Bosslet et al. 2015). If the patient in question meets the definition of "persistent" VS—a VS lasting a month or more, but not yet meeting the threshold for being considered chronic—then the patient has the potential for recovery under certain conditions (e.g., the patient doesn't have advanced dementia or other neurodegenerative disease and doesn't have other conditions likely to result in death in the near future). Dialysis is the treatment for renal disease and failure—it is effective whether or not the patient is conscious, so the judgment that it is potentially inappropriate does not depend on considerations of efficacy. Dialysis for this patient would presumably count as "potentially inappropriate" under the second criterion, where "there is no reasonable expectation that the patient's neurologic function will improve sufficiently to allow the patient to perceive the benefits of treatment." Yet this judgment explicitly must either rely on controversial quality of life judgments about what count as the "benefits of treatment," or on unattainable prognostic certainty concerning "sufficient" cognitive improvement, or both. There is ambiguity baked into terms like *reasonable expectation*, *sufficient* neurologic function, and *benefits of treatment*. To expand on the last two, whether an individual patient has sufficient neurologic function to perceive the benefits of treatment can depend a great deal on what benefits are under consideration. Benefits like reducing pain or having hedonic states minimally require sentience, but not sophisticated cognitive abilities. A benefit like continued life, on the other hand, might require fairly sophisticated cognitive abilities like self-awareness and awareness of the future. If we require having the ability to appreciate that benefit, we have to exclude a lot of people—infants, patients in the MCS, and people with some cognitive and intellectual disabilities. If that is the threshold, I think we set the bar too high. But appreciating the benefit of continued life could also mean appreciating the pleasures of the moment, pleasures only possible if one is alive. Terry Wallis reportedly has no sense of time—he is, for all he knows, still the 19-year-old man he was when his brain injury occurred—but he also knows that his "life is good."

5.5.3 Michael Hickson

In the summer of 2020, Michael Hickson, a 46-year-old father of five, was hospitalized with COVID-19 at St. David's Medical Center in Austin, Texas. Three years earlier, Hickson, an insurance claims estimator, was driving his wife Melissa to work when he suffered a sudden cardiac arrest. Paramedics resuscitated him, but the temporary loss of oxygen to his brain resulted in an anoxic brain injury, blindness, and quadriplegia.

On June 5, Melissa Hickson arrived at the hospital and was told that the medical staff had decided to stop treating her husband, would not put him on a ventilator, and would move him from the ICU to hospice. Melissa Hickson recorded a conversation with her husband's doctor, which was later posted to YouTube (Hickson 2020):

DOCTOR: "And the issue is, will this help him improve his quality of life? Cause as of right now, his quality of life . . . he doesn't have much of one."

MELISSA HICKSON: "What do you mean? Because he's paralyzed with a brain injury he doesn't have a quality of life?"

DOCTOR: "Correct."

The hospital argued that it was medically impossible to save Hickson, invoking physiological futility as a reason for denying Hickson the drug remdesivir and a life-saving ventilator. The doctor in the recording, however, appeared to view the use of a ventilator as "futile" because of Hickson's disability and his quality of life. According to Hickson's sister, a physician herself, Hickson could carry on a conversation, remember birthdays and his social security number, tell her about the foods he loved (gumbo and chocolate), help her pick out books to read, and report that he enjoyed the books. But he had no concept of time and couldn't formulate lists of common things like breakfast foods (Cha 2020). Hickson, in other words, while he had cognitive impairments, was a patient who appeared to have sufficient cognitive ability to appreciate his life and to appreciate the benefits of life-saving treatment.

Melissa Hickson told a reporter that if her husband had been asked if he wanted treatment, "He would say 'I want to live. I love my family and my children and they're the most important things to me.' He would probably say that's the reason for the past three years I have fought to survive" (Shapiro 2020).

Hickson did not survive his hospitalization. On the night of June 11, he died. The hospital notified his wife Melissa the following day.

One of the objectives of clarifying the concept of futility is to respond to ethical concerns about bias and subjectivity in using quality of life judgments to assess when treatment is futile or benefits the patient. These concerns have been frequently expressed by disability advocates and disabled persons, who claim that they are denied needed medical treatment because it is deemed futile due to preconceptions about their quality of life, or because a treatment will not affect their disability status. Shifting from "futility" to "potentially inappropriate" doesn't address those concerns, but instead introduces further ambiguity and value judgments, and counterproductively can have the effect of exacerbating distrust in medical providers. Steven Spohn, a disabled man, commented on

Hickson's case on Twitter: "We live our entire lives in fear that one day a doctor will decide we just aren't worth it" (Spohn 2020).

Appropriate uses of the concept of "potentially inappropriate intervention" are possible, but limited. In 1999, Sheila Pouliot was a 42-year-old developmentally disabled woman whose family sought to have all but pain treatment withdrawn as she lay dying in a hospital in Syracuse, New York. New York State law at the time prohibited the withdrawal of ANH (and continues to be particularly restrictive concerning withdrawal or withholding of ANH for developmentally disabled individuals). Due to Pouliot's medical condition, which included a nonfunctioning intestine and severe abdominal pain, the provision of nutrition, while it was not futile in the sense that it could not work, caused Pouliot "intense suffering with no corresponding medical benefits—beyond prolonging her life" (*Blouin v. Spitzer* 2002, Ouellette 2004). Pouliot's doctors judged treatment to be "medically inappropriate" and said it caused her "grotesque harm." A state supreme court judge, after visiting Pouliot's bedside, ordered the hospital to terminate ANH, saying "There's the law, and there's what's right" (Ouellette 2004). Indeed, because the treatment itself caused iatrogenic suffering—Pouliot experienced unrelievable pain and suffering—it was medically and ethically inappropriate.

Alicia Ouellette criticized New York's law at the time as "vitalism run amuck," and argued that it in essence forced treatment on incapacitated patients who may not have wanted it by taking away from their surrogates the power to act on their behalf (Ouellette 2004, 2006). This was especially true for patients who never had decisional capacity, such as those with developmental disabilities. But it applied as well to those with acquired brain injuries who did not, when they had decisional capacity, specifically document their preferences concerning future medical treatment.

One might also question whether Pouliot's treatment was inappropriate because she lacked sufficient cognitive ability to appreciate the benefits of treatment. That is the wrong question, and one that does not need an answer, because there were clear, ethical reasons to withdraw a harmful treatment. Pouliot was dying, and she was suffering as a direct result of LST.

Judgments about survival with sufficient cognitive ability are judgments about quality of life or about the value of a life, and they are potentially covert judgments about the value of an individual's life. Those kinds of contested and controversial judgments about the benefits of treatments that could work undermine trust when surrogates and patients disagree or suspect bias on the part of medical staff. The multi-society position paper stated that the ethical concerns that can justify treatment refusals on the part of physicians are that the treatment is "highly unlikely to be successful, is extremely expensive, or is intended to achieve a goal of controversial value" (Bosslet et al. 2015, 1322). Statements like that are why disabled persons worry that healthcare providers will conclude that their continued existence with a disability is not worth the expense or effort needed to keep them alive.

Ambiguous and poorly defined "ethical considerations" can easily turn into blatantly unethical considerations. Shifting conceptually from "futility" to "potentially inappropriate" doesn't successfully disambiguate the meaning of futility. Moreover, it continues to rely on contested judgments about quality of life and often assumes a level of prognostic certainty that is not attainable, and that cannot adequately support denials of treatments that could benefit patients.

5.6 Wicked Problems

The downstream risks or problems associated with brain injuries are complex. But they are more than just medically or ethically complex, because one aspect of these problems is that how the problems are formulated—their ontology—points us toward different potential solutions. Those solutions may lead to still other problems. For example, if we identify as a downstream problem the dearth of neurorehabilitative services available for patients with brain injuries, or the economic and financial burdens of caring for individuals with ongoing medical and rehabilitative needs, then resource-related solutions are called for to solve the problem so formulated. But that doesn't address a different problem: that some of those individuals might have lives that they don't wish to continue living. A problem framed that way might be addressed by changing laws concerning Medical Aid in Dying (MAiD), which is a logistically, legally, and socially complex downstream solution to a downstream problem. The risk inversion problem so framed is best addressed not through prevention, but by dealing with the downstream consequence—a life not worth living—if and when it arises. But that is not a suitable solution if the problem is instead framed as involving the misuse or waste of money or medical resources.

What I'm identifying as the risk inversion problem is the upstream foreclosing of options and opportunities for survival based on speculation about the risks of an uncertain, downstream future. But that is only one possible way to define the problem. If we identified it instead as a bean-counting problem, then by limiting treatment (and costs) upstream, we avoid future costs downstream—we reduce the use of financial and medical resources, and the resulting financial burdens. If we view the upstream/downstream problem as a problem of medical futility, then the upstream problem is using medical resources unwisely and unjustly, in a way that serves no good or desirable end. This way of looking at DoCs has been common since the early days and has flowed upstream to influence neurointensive care decisions. The neurointensive care environment provides the upstream solution to the downstream problem so conceived—death can come quickly and easily, avoiding a cursed survival. On this view, the upstream/downstream problem as I describe it isn't a problem at all. It's a solution.

The upstream problem as I frame it involves diagnostic and prognostic uncertainty coupled with social beliefs, values, and biases like ableism. Scientifically tackling the problem of diagnostic and prognostic uncertainty might not change upstream decisions at all—indeed, there might be even more epistemic confidence in those decisions to withhold treatment upstream, to avoid other, non-epistemic downstream risks. Some might think, for example, that being able to predict a prolonged recovery requiring intensive and expensive rehabilitation resources, rather than providing reasons against continuing intensive care treatment, provides financial, social, or even personal justifications for withdrawing LST early on. As in three-dimensional chess, moving a piece on one level changes the conflicts and possible moves on other levels.

Thus, different ways of formulating the problem imply different solutions and rule out other solutions. The upstream/downstream problem is akin to what are called "wicked problems" in social and policy planning. Rittel and Webber coined the term *wicked problems* in 1973 to describe incorrigible policy problems (Rittel and Webber 1973; Lavery 2018).[3] First, as described above, wicked problems are not amenable to definitive formulation. A wicked problem can be explained in numerous ways, and the framing determines potential solutions. "Unlike problems where there is little disagreement about its basic formulation, wicked problems are characterized by deep ambiguity in the ontological assumptions and metaphysical categories used in their articulation" (Whyte and Thompson 2012). The wicked problem at hand—risk inversion— can be explained by bean counting, the valorization of conscious life, ableism, medical futility (itself a wicked problem), or risk aversion. Second, there is no clearly foreseeable or obvious point

---

[3] In contrast to wicked problems are so-called tame problems, which are easily defined and solved. Some problems have been called "super wicked" because "time is running out, no one is in charge, those trying to solve the problems are causing them, and approaches have unknowable future consequences" (Conley et al. 2018). Conley et al. identified antibiotic resistance as a super wicked problem.

when we know the wicked problem will stop or be solved. Will it be when there is some threshold level of prognostic certainty in neurointensive care? Will it be when withdrawal of LST no longer occurs in neurointensive care? Both of these "stopping points" lead to other potential problems that are inseparable from the wicked problem, because, third, every wicked problem can be considered a symptom of another problem. Fourth, wicked problems are also characterized by there being no true or false solution, but rather solutions that are good or bad. But different stakeholders might view a solution as good or bad depending on their interests and their definition of the problem. Fifth, wicked problems also admit of many possible solutions, with no criteria for proving that every potential solution has been identified. Sixth, wicked problems are essentially unique, meaning that they have distinguishing properties that make them importantly unlike other, seemingly similar problems. The kinds of solutions we might apply to those seemingly similar problems will be incompatible with the wicked problem at hand. What was defined as the problem of DoCs in the 1970s—that we were pointlessly keeping hopeless cases alive—is solved by the very risk-inverting practices that constitute the current upstream/downstream problem.

Finally, and importantly for our discussion, the agents involved in wicked problems have no "right to be wrong." Their actions generate consequences that cannot be undone, "they leave permanent marks" (Whyte and Thompson 2012) for which the agents are liable, and "the effects can matter a great deal to those people touched by the actions" (Rittel and Webber 1973). Acting upstream has consequences for which those proposing solutions will be responsible. While neuroscientists can explore and experiment as they look to unlock the secrets of consciousness, placing patients into scanners to see what they can do, the neurointensivist who "applies a solution" to a wicked problem—what to do for this patient in this bed—isn't tinkering and doesn't have the luxury of consequence-free trial-and-error experimentation.

The upstream/downstream risk inversion problem is a wicked problem. It is difficult to formulate exactly what the problem is because it is partly constituted by epistemic uncertainty, and social, cultural, spiritual, individual, familial, financial, and political factors. It is not a problem with a straightforward solution or an obvious stopping point. It is not possible to achieve prognostic certainty for individual patients that is commensurate with the risks of different actions for individual patients. And individual preferences and tolerance for risk make one-size-fits-all policies onerous and ethically dodgy. Solutions are better or worse depending on individual consequences and circumstances, as well as contextual features that are beyond the control of the affected individuals.

5.7 Reinverting the Risks: Choosing Between Rocks and Hard Places

Wicked problems are notoriously unsolvable, or, at least, not completely solvable. We could, for example, reinvert the risks of withdrawing LST from patients in neurointensive care by not withdrawing LST. We could wait longer, until more epistemic certainty is possible. It may be months or years before that certainty is possible for DoC patients. The downstream risks, which are speculative, may or may not come to pass. This is not an entirely satisfactory solution, because if an unacceptable downstream consequence does come to pass, it will be bad for someone. The waiting may also be bad for someone (or multiple someones). We will have solved one problem by creating another, or others, which is one of the characteristics that make wicked problems so wicked and vexing.

Waiting longer in hopes of achieving more prognostic certainty runs the risk that some patients will survive in a condition they would judge undesirable or unacceptable. The solution to that problem could be to permit MAiD, but expanding access to that also carries ethical risks, particularly in this context, because many of those who will be "stuck" will not be able to make decisions for themselves. Should we maintain current constraints on assisted suicide (or euthanasia where it is permitted), for example, MaiD will be limited to those who have decisional capacity and can request it themselves, and that rules out DoC patients, and many others with brain injuries. Should we remove such limits and allow surrogates to make those choices, the ethical concerns that prompted those limits in the first place—that incapacitated patients will not be protected from decisions that are not in their interests and may be involuntarily killed—rise to the surface.

It can also be asked whether the apparent inversion of risks in withdrawing LST after brain injury actually involves a mistake. If one takes a vitalist position and views the continued biological life of a human as valuable, or perhaps of ultimate and immeasurable value, one might think it is a very serious mistake to allow that life to end when it could be saved. I do not hold that view. There might still be a mistake, however, in the comparing and weighing of the risks involved in continuing or discontinuing LST. As noted above, the risk inversion here is both ethical and epistemic. By choosing an epistemically certain but ethically risky outcome over an epistemically uncertain and ethically risky outcome, we create ethical risks that do not exist but for our choice.

The risk of dying if LST is withdrawn in neurointensive care is near 100 percent.[4] If some of the persons who died might have survived, and might have had on balance good lives that they valued, then we might well think that a significant opportunity was lost and a grave mistake was made. When the risk of surviving with an unacceptable life is perceived to be greater than the possibility of surviving to live a good and flourishing life, decision makers

---

[4] In the Ethicus Study of European ICUs and withdrawal of LST, 95.5 percent of patients died after treatment withdrawal. The study included a range of patients, not just brain injury patients. Of the 31,417 patients admitted to ICU during the study, 13.5 percent had limitations of LST (Sprung et al. 2003). In Turgeon et al.'s study of withdrawal of LST after severe TBI, no patients survived withdrawal (Turgeon et al. 2011).

might be making one of several epistemic mistakes that invert the upstream and downstream risks, including: (1) overestimating prognostic certainty or underestimating prognostic uncertainty (including predictions of death, survival, and impairment/disability); (2) overestimating the badness of life with impairments and disability; (3) misunderstanding the patient's desires and values; (4) being unduly influenced by, and thereby perpetuating, self-fulfilling prophecies.[5] These are all epistemic errors that occur in part because of the prevalence of uncertainty in situations where upstream treatment decisions are made, and made under time pressure. When epistemic errors have irrevocable consequences and can result in avoidable deaths, we tend to rightly think they are serious mistakes. The inferences involved in decision-making for patients with brain injuries involve considerable inductive risks— ethical risks involving potentially avoidable deaths. Ethical risks ought to be minimized.

Whether the risk inversion can be corrected is the question. Because this is a wicked problem, the possible solutions carry consequential risks of their own. It is less a matter of navigating through, and more a matter of choosing between, rocks and hard places, of which there are many. Addressing the hard place of epistemic errors and uncertainty requires that clinicians acknowledge the epistemic limitations of diagnosis and prognosis—and hold those limitations in tension with the need and desire of surrogates for information as they attempt to navigate a treacherous decisional landscape. It requires of clinicians and surrogates that they acknowledge and account for the rocks—their own implicit and explicit biases concerning what counts as a good life, or a life worth

---

[5] In the study by Turgeon et al., three reasons were identified to justify decisions to withdraw LST after brain injuries: (i) "poor chance of survival (according to the medical team)," (ii) "prognosis incompatible with the patient's wishes (as indicated by the next of kin)," and (iii) "poor long-term neurologic prognosis (as indicated by the medical team)" (Turgeon et al. 2011). These are all prognostic and uncertain, and (ii) and (iii) involve inductive predictions about future capacities and quality of life.

saving and living—at the same time that they try to do what is best for patients who have/had their own biases and preferences and conceptions of a life that is good. And it requires recognizing that avoiding outright the rocks and hard places downstream requires significant, perhaps disproportionate, upstream sacrifices.

6

The Ethics of Uncertainty

Let's assemble the pieces.

In the previous chapters, I describe the uncertainties concerning consciousness and unconsciousness and the role of inferences in diagnostic and prognostic uncertainty in disorders of consciousness. The concepts of inductive risk, risk inversion, and wicked problems help illuminate the ontological and epistemic nature of the clinical challenges associated with decision-making about disorders of consciousness (DoCs). Having got our arms partway around the problem, grasping the ethical implications and considerations remains.

Different people will have different beliefs about, and tolerances for, the risks associated with withdrawing or continuing life-sustaining treatment (LST), or surviving with a DoC or disability. *Who* is deciding or taking the risk matters. Our tolerance for the ethical risks can be higher—that is, we can tolerate more risk—if those facing the risks are deciding for themselves. This tolerance can be equally high whether it's the risk of dying when they could have lived or the risk of living when they would rather have died. In other words, we can, and we should, respect patient autonomy and self-determination even when we think that a person has decided wrongly, or imprudently, or with imperfect knowledge. In the case of individuals with brain injuries, those decisions would often have been made prior to their injury, when they lacked specific information about their future condition. Although we have good reason to think that many people are not well informed about brain injuries and DoCs and harbor implicit and explicit biases about DoCs and disability, respecting persons requires respecting their wishes and respecting their right to be wrong about what they would desire in some hypothetical future. In terms of epistemic and testimonial justice, we might be guilty of granting excess credibility to individuals concerning their self-knowledge. Credibility excess, like credibility deficits, can be unjust. But we ought to be more concerned about credibility deficits, where someone's testimony is given too little credibility, and a corresponding excess of credibility is given to someone else, where it is not warranted and where there are resulting testimonial harms. Persons presumptively know themselves and their own preferences better than others do. Concerning individual self-knowledge, then, we are warranted in giving credence to their expressed preferences, even at the risk of granting excess credibility, because doing so will not be unjust and we have other important reasons (like respecting their self-determination) for doing so.

Not all choose for themselves, and not all choose to choose for themselves. Matters become more complicated when it comes to surrogate decision makers, given that there can be a mismatch between their desires or their understanding of what patients would want and what the patients really would decide for themselves. Surrogates sometimes project their own values and wishes onto the patients for whom they are making decisions (Fagerlin et al. 2001). Surrogates can be susceptible to cognitive biases like framing affects and heuristics that make them vulnerable to manipulation (intended or not) by physicians (Feltz and Samayoa 2012; Barnato and Arnold 2013). Surrogates face fraught, emotionally difficult, and extremely consequential decisions when someone they care about has a serious brain injury. There can be no guarantees that their decisions will always be the ones the patient would (if they could) make for themselves. As a practical matter, this is another choice between rocks and hard places, between allowing surrogates and families to make decisions on behalf of patients they know and care about, or allowing a disinterested third party—a doctor, a judge, a court-appointed guardian—to make those decisions.[1] Many people have preferences about who they want to make decisions for them (Mirzaei, Milanifar, and Asghari 2011) and would prefer that such decisions either be left to people they know and trust, or they would wish to make those decisions themselves through advance directives (High 1990). We ought to also honor those preferences when they can be known.

As an ethical matter, while both patients and surrogates can make inferences that don't fully account for uncertainties in acute and chronic brain injuries and can be biased about quality of life, giving their authority to make ethically risky choices to a disinterested third party would violate the autonomy of patients, whether they have exercised that autonomy themselves through an advance directive or whether is it mediated through their surrogates. (In the case of M discussed below, it can be seen how disinterested third parties, like judges, are not really disinterested and can have their own biases.) In cultures where the expectation is that families make decisions on behalf patients, it would also constitute a violation of important and valuable cultural norms and traditions. Physicians and other medical staff who interact with patients and surrogates have their own implicit and explicit biases. Good shared decision-making demands that they give due weight to medical uncertainty and set aside their own subjective preferences and values in the interest of helping surrogates make decisions that are congruent with patient values and preferences whenever possible (Johnson and Cerminara 2020).

---

[1] I'm not suggesting here that family surrogates always *do* care about the patients they decide for. Families can become estranged, or have bad relationships, or conflicts of interests. When there are multiple and coequal surrogates, they can disagree about what to do.

6.1 Ethical Load Bearing: The Weight of Inference

The various problems and concerns discussed in previous chapters have practical consequences for individual patients. The first problem can be distilled to the Problem of Inductive Risk: Given uncertainty, what is the appropriate epistemic standard of evidence for accepting (and acting on) a diagnosis and/or prognosis? The First Principle of Inductive Risk provides this answer: The acceptable level of epistemic risk or uncertainty varies and should be limited by the ethical risks of being wrong. Where the ethical risks of being wrong are very serious, like avoidable deaths or survival with a life not worth living, we rightly demand a high level of certainty. But there remains an important question: How ought we respond in our ethical decision-making to uncertainty? And there the Second Principle of Inductive Risk provides an answer: The acceptable level of ethical risk varies and should be limited by the level of epistemic uncertainty. That is, we ought to take fewer or smaller ethical risks when faced with a lot of epistemic uncertainty. Both the First and Second Principles index risk to uncertainty. The First indexes epistemic risk-taking and the acceptance of uncertainty to ethical risks, while the Second indexes ethical risk-taking to epistemic uncertainty. Neither principle is a method for quantifying uncertainty and risk. The badness of specific risks (e.g., death, pain) is obvious but only subjectively quantifiable. Neither the First nor the Second Principle alone provides very specific answers to the question that matters a great deal in the context of brain injuries and DoCs: What is the right thing to do for this patient? Principles are like that. They trade in generalities rather than specifics.

Inferences also trade in generalities. Inferences about behavior and consciousness consider what is typical—what we would expect a typically functioning human to do when presented with a stimulus or when given a command. Inferences about brain behaviors also look at what is typical, averaging the results from healthy subjects to create a general map of brain activations in response to different stimuli.[2] When a subject with atypical outward behaviors has a brain that responds in ways that closely overlap the map, consciousness is inferred. At the level of specific, individual decision-making, the overarching medical and ethical conundrums turn on how much weight to give to diagnostic and prognostic inferences concerning brain injuries and DoCs. An unhelpfully nonspecific answer provided by the Second Principle is: the amount commensurate with their accuracy and certainty.

The prescription to index ethical and epistemic risks applies to knowers—physicians, medical staff, bioethicists, and others in a position of having and transmitting clinical knowledge—who counsel patients and patient surrogates. It also applies to societies and social communities—to everyone who shapes policies and public attitudes. It is rightly a part of every conversation, formal or informal, about advance directives. The decisions about what ought to be done for and about DoC patients are not entirely unique—similar decisions are made every day in the face of uncertainty, for children with cancer, for extremely premature neonates, for 20-year-old warfighters with devastating injuries, for elderly patients with dementia, and many others. But to be clear, when surrogates face an agonizing decision concerning a specific patient, someone they care about, the onus is on the medical staff they interact with to do the calculating and to provide them with the relevant, relative uncertainties and risks. Surrogates are in the best position to know how the patient might weigh uncertainty and can choose how to incorporate that uncertainty into the complex, multifactorial array of information and interests that shapes their decisions, but their epistemic obligations are less demanding. Ideally, surrogates would and could optimize the balance of epistemic and ethical risks as

---

[2] Interestingly, because there can be anatomical differences between the brains of right-handed and left-handed people, many brain-mapping projects use only right-handed subjects.

they confront uncertainties and the need to make choices. But in ideal circumstances, epistemic and ethical uncertainty would not exist. In the non-ideal world in which highly personal, emotional, and difficult decisions must be made under conditions of some-times brutal uncertainty, the obligations of surrogates are to make decisions that are uncertainly right or best, all things considered. They must make decisions they, and the patients they decide for, can live with. That sometimes means choosing against continuing life for the patient who faces a future they can't, or won't want to, live with. And sometimes it means choosing to continue treatment.

6.2   Universal Moral Prescriptions

In chapter 2, I discuss the way that *vegetative* functions as a thick concept, one that is not merely descriptive, but also prescriptive. There have been, throughout the history of the vegetative state/un-responsive wakefulness syndrome (VS/UWS)—and similarly the minimally conscious state (MCS)—numerous attempts to draw out universal moral conclusions and prescriptions concerning patients. These include judgments that unconscious humans are no longer persons, no longer alive, and not entitled to life-sustaining treat-ment, as well as judgments concerning what is in the "best interests" of unconscious humans. Early on, legal, ethical, and medical con-sensus coalesced around the view that it was not in the interests of unconscious patients, or society, to keep them alive indefinitely. There were, of course, always minority reports, arguments against stripping these patients of their humanity and their rights to life and medical treatment.

As more is learned about DoCs and DoC patients, in particular the diversity of these patients and the varied expressions of these disorders, such universal prescriptions have become increasingly outdated, untenable, unhelpful, and un-useful. There are several reasons for this. One is the epistemic uncertainty of consciousness and unconsciousness. Even if it is accepted that moral personhood depends on consciousness—a suspect premise at best—ethical conclusions about the moral personhood of an individual can be no more certain than epistemic conclusions about their consciousness. And at present, and for several decades now, those diagnostic and prognostic conclusions have been wrong for 4 in 10 cases. Are unconscious individuals alive? Again, even if we accept the ontological premise that being a living person requires consciousness and a functioning neocortex, we can expect to stumble on the epistemic, on the actual verification of who is and who is not a living person. Whether unconscious persons are entitled to LST is a properly ethical, rather than ontological, question. Applying the Second Principle of Inductive Risk and indexing the ethical risk of denying LST to the epistemic risk of being wrong about unconsciousness tells us that ethically fraught decisions to forgo the possibility of surviving with a good-enough life require a level of epistemic certainty that is not met.

The entangled uncertainties here—the ontological, epistemic, and ethical—are such that, even if we could diminish or eliminate uncertainty in one realm, we would still be left with uncertainties in the others. Suppose, for example, we developed the ability to accurately diagnose what currently counts as consciousness in the clinical realm, reducing our false negatives to a clinically acceptable level. There would remain ontological uncertainty: Is this thing we call consciousness actually consciousness? Is it the relevant kind of consciousness? And there would remain ethical uncertainty: Is consciousness necessary for an entity to matter morally? In what way do conscious entities matter? What are our moral obligations to conscious entities?

And then there will be still other questions at the level of individual patients. For determinations about what is in the best interests of DoC patients, there is no defensible answer that applies universally across all patients, or across the existing classifications of DoCs. While there is a reasonable question as to whether an unconscious being can have interests at all, answering that question is complicated by the subjective nature of well-being, the possibility of interests that survive the loss of consciousness, and the social entanglement and embeddedness of human interests. When it comes to our interests, we are not islands, free-floating and unconnected to the interests of others in our families, social circles, and communities.

In sum, universal moral prescriptions concerning what should be done for, or about, all DoC patients, or the moral status of all DoC patients (or all VS/UWS patients, all MCS patients, etc.), to the extent that they are grounded in consciousness/unconsciousness, are at best on ground too unstable to support them.

6.3 Moral Prescriptions

One might throw one's hands up at this point and conclude that epistemic uncertainty is fatal to ethical decision-making on behalf of DoC patients, or in any context where there is a lot of uncertainty. Moreover, the context of DoCs is one of triple jeopardy, in which there is also ontological uncertainty. But decision-making for patients with brain injuries and DoCs is unavoidable, not just in the immediate aftermath of injury, but at all points in their lives post-injury. Likewise for every patient who lacks the capacity to decide for themselves and direct their own care and treatment, and those who never had the capacity, including infants, children, and some persons with cognitive or intellectual disabilities. So, since we must make decisions, and throwing up our hands is not an option, the task is to determine how, and how best, to do it.

The framework of core ethical principles commonly employed in medical ethics provides a starting point. Respect for persons and their autonomy, beneficence/nonmaleficence, and justice are generally considered to be nonhierarchical principles—none is more important, and none takes precedence over the others. Except that

it is not at all unusual for the attempted deployment of these principles to result in conflicts, at which point, one must choose.

6.3.1 Autonomy and Respect for Persons

In Western medical contexts, priority is frequently given to respect
for individual patient autonomy. As noted above, however, not
everyone for whom decisions must be made was at some point in
their lives autonomous in the way required for medical decision-
making, that is, having the capacity to make decisions and provide informed consent, and being capable of self-determination
and self-rule. Additionally, some religious communities and non-
Western cultures and communities value individual autonomy less
than family or collective decision-making, and so we ought not insist that there is a single ideal—respecting individual autonomy—
that solves all our problems.

It does solve some problems, just in case respecting the patient's
wishes and values was/is important to the patient, and the patient
left enough information to go on for the decision at hand. An advance directive or similar document can provide evidence of both,
because we can conclude that the patient wanted to direct their own
care and treatment enough to put it in writing. Ideally, the directives
are specific enough to guide decisions in the situation at hand. But
that is where things get messy. Advance directives are often quite
general and lack the specificity we'd like to have to be confident that
they fit the context. So, must we apply and interpret them?

We must. The moral justification for respecting patient
preferences and choices regarding treatment is that individuals
value self-determination and self-rule. Violations of individual
self-rule in the form of forced or unwanted treatment impinge on,
and injure, bodily liberty and sovereignty, and the security of the
person, and deprive patients of their right of self-determination.
The importance of respecting self-determination is also grounded

in the epistemic view that individuals know best what is in their own interests and what accords with their own values. Thus, respecting individual self-determination is also a matter of epistemic justice. All this has the salutary effect of protecting those with unconventional views—those who might be seen as acting or choosing against their own interests—as well as those with more mainstream views about what is good and valuable. It also protects those who are vulnerable to others' misinterpretations of the value or quality of their lives. It is presumed that individual values inform preferences, and that not everyone has the same values when it comes to illness, injury, or death. Some individuals would prefer death to being permanently disabled. Others would rather die than violate their religious beliefs. And some believe that when and whether they die is not a matter to be decided by human or medical intervention. The moral imperative to respect individual autonomy remains even if the individual's values and preferences appear peculiar, imprudent, baffling, or misinformed, and even if their choices are incongruent with someone else's notion of their best interests or welfare. The right of self-determination does not require the approval of others.

It is, of course, very difficult for surrogates at times to enact the will of an incapacitated patient. There can be interpretive uncertainty about what the patient really wants and under what circumstances. There can be uncertainty about whether they suffer, whether this is the kind of life they would want, and what is in their best interests. Some patients may have only casually discussed their preferences with family or confidants, or they may have spoken in broad generalities about not wanting to be "hooked up to tubes and machines." Some have said nothing at all. Among patients who have previously expressed their preferences, few have considered liminal states like the MCS, or considered uncertainty and the quantity of uncertainty they find acceptable. There are uncertainties about prognosis and diagnosis with brain injuries and DoCs, about quality of life (both immediately and in the long term), and about an individual's current needs, preferences, and desires, if they have any. Surrogates may frequently lack both relevant evidence about the patients' own wishes and lack certainty about what might be in their best interests, all things considered.

6.3.1.1 Robert Wendland

> *"Just let me go."*
>
> —Robert Wendland

Decision-making for patients in the MCS can be especially fraught because these patients are conscious and sentient. They may have current interests and desires but lack the capacity to express them. On September 29, 1993, Robert Wendland, a 41-year-old father, husband, and auto parts salesman, flipped his Dodge Ram truck. He was intoxicated and not wearing a seatbelt. He was thrown from his truck and sustained injuries that resulted in right-sided paralysis. He was comatose for 16 months, and for the next several years was in a condition described as "minimally conscious."[3] He could perform simple tasks with repetitive prompting, such as catching a ball. His wife and children believed he did not recognize them.

Two years after his accident, and after Wendland's feeding tube had been dislodged for the fourth time, his wife Rose sought to have tube feeding withdrawn permanently. Wendland's mother, Florence Wendland, objected, and a protracted legal battle followed, pitting different factions of the family against each other. Rose Wendland and her children all testified that Wendland had made his wishes clear—wishes he expressed after the death of his father-in-law—that he would not want to be kept alive in his present condition. Only days before his accident, he told his wife

---

[3] The MCS was not formally defined until the year after Wendland's death (Giacino et al. 2002).

"Don't let that happen to me. Just let me go." Rose described her husband's life as a "living hell" (Chiang 2001).

Wendland's case went to court. The judges expressed concerns that he might wish to live but was unable to affirm that wish. Wendland, who was capable of answering some yes/no questions (although it was unclear if he actually answered them deliberately, or merely randomly), had been asked if he wanted to die, but he did not answer the question. There are a number of reasons why someone in an MCS would not answer such an important question, but given that he was incapacitated and would not have met a legal standard of competence, it's unclear what possible purpose would be served by even asking Wendland the question. The judges gave great weight to the possibility that he wanted to live, although there was no way to confirm it in his case. Eventually, one judge ruled that although he had a "strong suspicion" that Wendland would have wanted to die under the circumstances, the evidence of his wishes was not strong enough under governing law to support termination of LST (Eisenberg and Kelso 2002). The sought-after standard of evidence was what the *Wendland* court described as "an exact 'on all fours' description of [his] present medical condition" (Johnson and Cerminara 2020). In this and other cases involving MCS patients, courts "did not accept as decisive statements about more vague conditions and treatments, spoken in the language people usually use when talking with friends and family about these decisions" (Johnson and Cerminara 2020).

Wendland died of pneumonia in July 2001, a month before the final court ruling was handed down in his case.

Because patients in the MCS are potentially capable of experiencing pain and other aversive states that might make their lives, on balance, worse than the lives of patients in the VS/UWS, limiting their right to refuse LST, although motivated by an abundance of caution, is potentially harmful in multiple ways. It may be physically and psychologically harmful, and also a violation of their rights as patients to refuse unwanted treatment. While patients in the MCS cannot exercise their autonomy, one of the roles of surrogates is to exercise it for them. Thwarting a surrogate in their fulfillment of that duty thwarts the self-determination of the patient as well.

In the VS/UWS and MCS, patients are unable to meaningfully communicate their current desires and preferences, if indeed they have any. Their previously expressed preferences are then, as it were, preserved in amber. If we are concerned that those stilled preferences do not reflect their current wishes or did not anticipate their current condition, then we might legitimately wonder if they should guide treatment and nontreatment decisions. Similar concerns have been raised about preferences that have been formally documented in advance directives, and not just those informally expressed to friends and family. For example, there is ongoing debate about whether the advance directives of persons with advanced dementia ought to apply after they lose decisional capacity. Should a previous treatment refusal that could result in death be honored if the patient seems content in their present condition? Ought a desire for all possible treatment be honored if the patient appears miserable or continued treatment might cause iatrogenic harms and suffering? Prior wishes ought to carry considerable weight—consistent with the intentions of the patient. There is a need for nuanced and thoughtful decision-making in such cases, and not just doctrinaire adherence to prior expressions, given the nonspecificity of many advance directives. That complicates, rather than simplifies, decision-making, which at this point should not surprise the reader.

6.3.2 Beneficence, Nonmaleficence, and Best Interests

As Robert Wendland's case demonstrates, when a patient in a chronic DoC is incapacitated and there is epistemic uncertainty about what they want, did want, or would want, what they are experiencing, and what lies ahead for them, there is also ethical uncertainty about what is in the patient's interests, including about how and where the patient should reside or receive care, and whether and for how long LST should continue. That is, there are questions about balancing the possible benefits and harms the patient might experience and, all things considered, what is in the patient's interests, or their best interests.

Dan Brock argued that irreversibly unconscious patients can have no interests, because having interests requires consciousness:

> If you were to suffer such severe brain damage as to leave you in a persistent vegetative state, would you still have an interest in measures aimed at sustaining or extending your life, or would continued life-sustaining measures no longer be of any interest or benefit for you? I believe that nearly all persons who reflect on this question conclude that because complete and permanent loss of consciousness carries with it the loss of all possibilities for agency and experience of any sort, continuing to sustain the life of the patient's body is of no benefit whatever to the patient. However the complex notion of interests is analyzed, it is usually concluded that a thing's having interests of its own in some object or state of affairs x is tied to the thing's present or future capacity for sentience and to its capacity to care about x. (1988, 80)

To be sure, a truly unconscious patient cannot have current *experiential* interests. They neither suffer nor enjoy their lives, nor the things that happen to them and around them. They do not, as Brock noted, care about any object or state of affairs. But the conclusion that they have no interests at all is wrong. If I am unconscious and under anesthesia, I am presumably feeling and experiencing nothing—neither positive nor aversive states. Nonetheless, I have an interest in the skill of the surgeon and the anesthesiologist, and in the successful outcome of my surgery.

If those kinds of interests do not seem nonsensical or impossible when I am temporarily unconscious under anesthesia, then neither should the interests I have if I am comatose following a brain injury. I have an interest in surviving, in recovering consciousness, in recovering from my injuries, and in my life being restored to what it was before (assuming I valued my life as it was before). And if I am in a chronic VS/UWS, it still makes sense that I could have those same interests. I can, if I am unconscious for some reason, also have interests in certain life plans of mine. I have projects and goals, things I'd like to do and see. But I can also have an interest in *not* living the kind of life where none of those things is possible for me. And so, I might have an interest in not living a life in which I am in constant pain, or in which I will never regain consciousness, never be able to converse with another person, or pet a dog, or eat a delicious meal, or swim in a warm, turquoise sea. I might have an interest in what happens to my family, whether caring for me will burden them or cause them to suffer. The point is that VS/UWS patients do have interests in states of affairs, even if they are unaware and unable to conceive of, or have desires about, or think about, those states of affairs and their interests right now. And if they have interests, like you and me, then we can assume they could also have best interests, like you and me. If only we could know what they are.

But, you might be thinking, someone who will never regain consciousness will never be able to conceive of, or think about, or feel anything about, anything, including their interests. Their interests are simply gone, along with their consciousness. Again, that strikes me as wrong. They can still have interests, just as I can when I'm under anesthesia. That one of us is more likely to wake up and be capable of acting in our own interests (or changing them in the course of our lives) is beside the point (and if it isn't, I've yet to see an argument explaining how it is not beside the point). We endeavor to act in the interests of unconscious patients all the time—when we enact their advance directives and preferences, when we make decisions on their behalf that are in their best interests (as Nancy Cruzan's family tried to do). Nancy Cruzan's father Lester Cruzan said:

> If they really cared about Nancy the way we do, they would want to turn her loose. I know damn well if it were me up there I would be furious with the state of Missouri because of what they had done to my family by forcing me to stay alive. And I feel very much Nancy would feel the same way, because Nancy cared very dearly for her family. (Quoted in Robbins 1989)

There is nothing incoherent about Lester Cruzan's statement. It expresses how Nancy would feel and what she would want—it is a coherent expression of her interests in her family and in the kind of life she would want to live. If we truly thought that unconscious individuals no longer had any interests at all, we would be hard pressed to make decisions on their behalf that protect, or act in, their (nonexistent) interests. It would be incoherent for a father to say of his daughter that she would not want to be kept alive.

MCS patients are conscious but may not have the kinds of current interests that they can hold in mind and think about, interests in life plans and goals and projects. We might think they are similar to infants, with experiences and experiential interests. What is in their best interests, then, is likely to be similar to the best interests of those in the VS/UWS, except that MCS patients might also experience pleasures and pains, as well as positive and negative emotional states. Patients in the MCS exist on a spectrum of awareness and functioning, each one living in a state of flux, with potentially some comprehension and perceptual awareness. That is, MCS patients might also have current, experiential interests, just as infants do, but lack the ability to unambiguously express them. This was the concern expressed by the judges in *Wendland*.

Given that they have interests, it is possible to act beneficently and nonmaleficently toward DoC patients. We can do right and wrong by them, even if they are not aware of what we do. The ways we can do right and wrong by them are the same ways we do right and wrong by other persons. We might misdiagnose them, leading to a cascade of other possible harms. We might cause some of them pain or distress. We might violate their rights by subjecting them to unwanted treatment, or by denying them treatment they want (or wanted). We might force them to continue living when they are powerless to stop us. We might terminate their lives by withdrawing treatment when they are powerless to stop us. We might subject them to burdens that, on balance, and for them, outweigh the benefits. We might assign them less value than other humans, write them off as lost causes, medically and socially neglect them, and expel them from our communities and webs of concern. We might also do right by them when we respect their preferences, as we understand them, and treat them as persons with rights—rights to exist and live, and a right to choose their own death.

6.3.2.1 M

In the United Kingdom, decisions to withdraw LST from DoC and other incapacitated patients must be approved by courts, although in most cases it is a mere formality. Withdrawal is rarely denied for patients in the VS/UWS or MCS. The ethical and legal standard used to justify these decisions is the "best interests" standard. Under the Mental Capacity Act of 2005, a conclusion about best interests is arrived at by balancing the benefits and burdens of their life (a process that is described as literally drawing up a balance sheet) alongside consideration of the patient's past wishes, and the sanctity of life. For patients in the VS/UWS, "the prevailing assumption is that life-prolonging treatment is not in their best interests because it is futile" (Jackson 2013). Justices have acknowledged the tension in using the best interests standard in VS/UWS cases, tension that is supposedly resolved by admitting that they cannot have interests in either continuing or terminating LST, as expressed by the House of Lords in the case concerning Tony Bland:

The distressing truth which must not be shirked is that the proposed conduct is not in the best interests of Anthony Bland, for he has no best interests of any kind. . . . Although the termination of his life is not in the best interests of Anthony Bland, his best interests in being kept alive have also disappeared.

It must be a matter of complete indifference whether he lives or dies. (Lords Mustill and Keith, in *Airedale NHS Trust v. Bland*, quoted in Jackson 2013)

This valiant attempt to square the circle concludes that if an individual has no interests at all, it is not in their interests to continue LST. The futility (or lack of benefit) of the treatment (tube feeding, in Bland's case) tips the balance against continuing. This is, in essence, an argument frequently made concerning withdrawal of LST from unconscious patients in the VS/UWS: (1) they derive no benefit, (2) they have no interests, and (C) it is therefore not possible that it is in their interests to continue LST. As I argue above, I think the second premise can be challenged, and without it, the conclusion cannot stand. We should also, at this moment in time (but perhaps not when the Bland decision was rendered) be skeptical about the certainty of unconsciousness in at least some cases.

In the case of *W v M*, involving a patient in the MCS, the Court of Protection denied the request to withdraw LST. The case is considered an anomaly and has been widely criticized as incorrectly decided.[4]

On February 17, 2003, M, then age 43, went to bed early with a headache. She was set to leave the following day for a ski trip. When she didn't get out of bed early, as was her habit, her longtime partner (known as S in the court proceedings quoted below) checked on her and found her in a drowsy and confused state. She was taken to hospital and fell into a coma. She had contracted viral encephalitis, which left her with extensive neurological damage. She was

---

[4] Personal communication with Celia Kitzinger.

diagnosed in a VS after emerging from coma. In 2007, her family applied for a court order authorizing the withdrawal of artificial nutrition and hydration (ANH). The court-ordered assessment eventually concluded that M was in the MCS, but that "there was a possibility that she was in fact at a higher level of function than she was at that time demonstrating."

> It is clear to me that M has a high[er] level of responses than pre-
> viously identified. Because of the lack of consistency and the ina-
> bility to use them, as yet, for communication purposes, this places
> her in the diagnostic category of minimally conscious state—but
> at a moderate level of MCS. I say moderate level to indicate that
> these are not simple responses but are indicating some sophistica-
> tion in the response level. . . . In summary, it is clear to me that she
> is NOT in the vegetative state. Moreover, she is making responses
> at a level that must raise the possibility that she will eventually
> be able to communicate. In view of this, it is my opinion that she
> requires the opportunity of access to a team very experienced in
> the assessment or management of people with this level of pro-
> found neurological disability. (Dr. Keith Andrews, quoted in *W
> v M* 2011)

Rehabilitation, rather than withdrawal of LST, was recommended. Two years later, in 2009, M was assessed by Lynne Turner-Stokes, whose view of M's capacities was less optimistic, as reported by Baker J ("Baker J" refers to The Honorable Mr. Justice Baker, fol-lowing the citation conventions used in the United Kingdom):

> She stated that she was unable to identify any aspect of M's life
> that gave her positive pleasure or satisfaction. On the contrary,
> Professor Turner-Stokes concluded that M had marked hyper-
> sensitivity and was experiencing a significant level of discomfort
> and, on occasions, pain. She confirmed that there was no real-
> istic possibility of recovery and concluded that, in her opinion, it

would be appropriate to withdraw artificial nutrition and hydration to allow M to die in dignity.

M's family again petitioned for withdrawal of ANH. Per the United Kingdom's Mental Capacity Act of 2005, "Any decision made under the Mental Capacity Act for a person who lacks capacity must be made in her best interests. The law requires the court to identify those factors which are relevant to the person's best interests and carry out a balancing exercise weighing up the factors on each side of the issue" (*W v M* 2011). *W v M* was the first case considered by the Court of Protection involving the withdrawal of LST from a patient in the MCS.

M's sister "B" testified that M would not want to be kept alive in her present condition, and that she would not want to live in a nursing home.

> B described how M had firm views on many things. Both of them had been very close to their maternal grandmother who in her nineties had gone to live in a nursing home where her health and capacity had gradually declined. B recounted that M had always said that, if she was in danger of going into residential home, she would rather shorten her life by ten years rather than have someone look after her. B told me that M did not wish to be looked after in the way that her grandmother had been. She was fiercely independent and according to B would have hated to have been looked after. B described how M had said similar things when their father became ill a few years later and had to go into a care home and also during the time of the publicity about the Tony Bland case.
>
> B stressed that she could not argue with the quality of care that M has received in her nursing home. Her argument was that she knew that M would not have wanted to live like this. B spoke how M was unable to move, speak or communicate with anyone. "Not to be able to communicate with anyone is inconceivable." She

accepted that M was able to open her eyes but asked: "Why is that meaningful?"

In oral evidence, B asked rhetorically: "What can she possibly get out of life? No pleasure. The daily routine of being got out of bed, put back, dressed, doubly incontinent. It's not a life, it's an existence and I know she wouldn't want it. It pains me every time to see her in bed, in the chair, she doesn't resemble anything she used to look like." B insisted that she was pursuing this application out of love for her sister. "It's solely for my sister. It would be easy to walk away but I'm here because I think I'm doing the right thing. I know that's what she wanted in her hearts of hearts." (*W v M* 2011)

Caregivers in M's nursing home described her responsiveness, which included opening her eyes when overhearing gossip and moving her hands and smiling when listening to music. She was described as moaning frequently, with different kinds of moans that her caregivers interpreted as expressing different needs and desires. She occasionally spoke intelligibly. Some descriptions of her emotional responses are quite poignant:

On one occasion in the summer of 2010, when M was in the living room, an Elvis Presley ballad was played on the television. C recalled looking at M and seeing tears rolling down her cheeks. That is the only occasion when she has seen M cry in response to music and thereafter she has taken care to avoid playing any Elvis songs. C described how on two occasions she has seen M cry after S has left the bedroom following a visit. On both occasions, M made no noise, but she can see tears rolling down her cheeks.

C gave evidence about how she had heard M talk on two different occasions. On the first occasion, whilst she and another carer were working together and were about to turn M over to change her, she said "bloody hell." More recently, on 12 April 2011, when she went in to see M early in the morning, she noticed that M was staring at her and she said "Good Morning" to which M replied, "what." C says that she repeated "Good Morning" to which M said "what." C then asked M if she was hot, to which M replied "yes." C then asked her if she wanted to take her blankets off, to which M replied "no." At this point, according to C, another carer came into the room called X. At this point, C crouched down to look directly at M and said, "Are you going to say good morning to X?" M replied "morning." At this point, according to C, M had both her eyes open. C says that she is absolutely clear that M spoke these words which were very distinct and clear. Cross-examined by Mr. Sachdeva, C insisted that it was not possible that she had misheard what M had said. She was quite taken aback because this had never happened before. This is the only occasion on which she has heard M apparently speak. C said that she had never seen M smile. In cross-examination, she said that it was "really hard" to say if M took pleasure in anything.

M's caregivers reported that she experienced pain, discomfort, or distress 25 to 30 percent of the time. Her family members argued that it was more frequent. Baker J concluded that she was not in "constant pain" nor was she in "extreme pain," that the absence of pain and discomfort had to be counted as "a positive feature of life," that "M does enjoy some aspects of her life," and that her experiences are not "on balance, negative." In deciding against the withdrawal of ANH, Baker J utilized the "balance sheet" approach, weighing positive against negative in M's life. He gave greater weight to the opinions of M's caregivers than to family evidence of M's previously expressed wishes:

I heard evidence from B and S, who spoke movingly about M and contrasted her previous life with her current circumstances. They told me about things that M had said before her collapse which, they maintain, demonstrated that she would not want to be kept alive in this condition. I also heard evidence from a number of members of the dedicated team of professional care staff, skills workers and physiotherapists who look after M in her present nursing home. They portrayed her life in much more positive terms [than] those used by members of her family. (*W v M* 2011)

Ultimately, what tipped the balance was "the importance of preserving life," which Baker J called "the decisive factor in this case," deciding that it was clear that "it would not be in M's best interests for ANH to be withdrawn." Baker J noted that testimonial reports of M's prior wishes were discounted, and

that an advance decision must address specifically the circumstances in which it will be binding and is made in the knowledge that it will be decisive if those circumstances arise. . . . There is no evidence that M ever specifically considered the question of withdrawal of ANH, or ever considered the question whether she would wish such treatment to be withdrawn if in a minimally conscious state.

This is essentially like the "exact on all fours" standard that the *Wendland* court specified, which imposes a nearly impossible requirement that is not consistent with the way people actually talk about their wishes, nor even how they express them formally in advance directives. M became ill almost exactly a year after the paper formally defining the MCS was published. It is unlikely that she would have known about the MCS, and it is impossible that years earlier, when she expressed her wishes while discussing her grandparents and Tony Bland, that she could have foreseen a future in which she would be in the MCS.

The court's decision is also internally incoherent. On the one hand, it discounts any interests M might have once had in how her life goes, or how she dies—interests that she conceivably still has—giving more weight to her possible current interests in continuing to live, or in the possibility that she changed her mind. As

M's lawyer argued, this is "fatal to giving substantial weight to M's previous or likely views . . . [and] no advance decision could ever be upheld, on the basis that [the patient] could have changed his or her mind" (*W v M* 2011). Indeed, it implies that advance directives should never be honored just in case the patient has changed their mind. The court's response—that a sufficiently specific advance directive, made in the knowledge that it would be binding, would stand—does not address the question. Whether something is spoken or put in writing, and whether a person really meant it or not, and whether they intended to bind themselves in the future or not, has no bearing whatsoever on the possibility that they later changed their mind. If that mere possibility—or uncertainty—carries a lot of weight, it will tip the balance against doing what the patient, in the past, said they would want done.

If "preservation of life" is given substantial weight—as it was in M's case—the balance will always tip in favor of the continuation of LST, because the patient's expressed wishes will have been discounted. That is, if the patient's past preferences were for continuation of LST, that plus the value of preserving life will tip in favor of LST; if the patient's past preferences were against LST, discounting those preferences on the chance that the patient changed their mind, plus the added weight given to preserving life, will tip the balance in favor of LST. If *W v M* served as a precedent for other cases involving MCS, it would seem impossible to withdraw LST from MCS patients, regardless of what those patients themselves would have wanted. Importantly, not everyone would agree that preserving life should have overriding or "added weight" value in considerations about their own fate, so a default to "preservation of life" might well conflict with an individual's own values in an objectionable way.

In M's case, there was disagreement about the balance of pleasure and pain she experienced. There was agreement that she experienced pain and discomfort every day—perhaps 25 to 30 percent of the time—but disagreement about whether she experienced any pleasures. Part of what makes MCS cases particularly difficult is that the patients are sentient but incapable of unambiguous communication. The meaning of M's moans, her bouts of crying, her facial expressions that might have been smiles and might have been grimaces, must be considered in the context of cognitive and motor impairments and the necessity of interpretations that are vulnerable to bias. There was, thus, considerable uncertainty about M's quality of life, and about what was in her best interests. But there was no disagreement—no uncertainty—among her family and partner about M's values and preferences, and about what she would want.

I have argued that DoC patients have enduring interests in what happens to them, in how their lives go, and that includes an interest in having their preferences and values honored. It is in the interests of DoC patients that their surrogates do what they would want them to do—to exercise their autonomy for them—and that remains true whether that means prolonging their lives or not. While the "preservation of life" is a value that is widely held and important, it's not life itself that is valuable and must be preserved—that would be mere vitalism. What M cared about, and what her surrogates cared about, was how her life fit the contours of what she considered a good, valuable, and meaningful life. It is in her interests to live (or die) in a way that conforms to her own values and preferences, not those of a judge.

Baker J affirmed that had M remained in the VS, the withdrawal of ANH would have been approved: "In VS cases, the balance falls in one direction in *every* case—in favor of withdrawal" (emphasis added; *W v M* 2011). Yet, nothing changed about M's life in the several years it took for her legal case to be brought to its conclusion—only the diagnosis changed. Thus, if it had been in her best interests to withdraw ANH in 2007, then all else being equal, it was in her best interests to withdraw ANH in 2011. But all else was not equal: the MCS diagnosis affirms the possibility not only that M was experiencing pain and distress, but also that she had some level of awareness of her condition, which could itself be a source of psychological distress. It would be reasonable to conclude that a sentient MCS patient, who can experience pain, discomfort, and distress (as M reportedly did) has a stronger claim to withdrawal of ANH than an unconscious patient who can feel nothing. That the right to refuse treatment and the right to die are denied to MCS patients on the grounds that they might have changed their minds threatens their autonomy rights, along with those of all other patients who lose their decisional capacity (Johnson 2011).

6.3.2.2 Persistent Uncertainties

Even if we accept that interests disappear along with permanent loss of consciousness (but not temporary loss of consciousness), and that the kind of enduring interests individuals have in how their lives go evaporate as well, we will still stumble on the epistemic uncertainty of unconsciousness, on high rates of misdiagnosis, on prognostic uncertainty, and on unknown numbers of potential patients with cognitive motor dissociation (CMD)—patients who are conscious, who have current experiences, and who have unknown and unrecognized interests, including interests in continuing, or not continuing, to live. If we acknowledge those uncertainties, we must also acknowledge that there is epistemic uncertainty about the existence and content of the interests of all DoC patients.[5] Does that give us a reason to assign more weight to those interests we can be certain about? I think it does. As a matter of epistemic justice, we ought to take seriously the preferences, wishes, and values of patients as they expressed them—however they expressed them—when they had capacity. We ought to take seriously the views of those who speak

[5] Brock, writing in 1988, dismissed concerns about misdiagnosis: "It would appear then, that the only self-regarding interest a person might have in continued life-sustaining treatment . . . is based on the possibility that the diagnosis and prognosis are mistaken and the condition is not irreversible. However, as the probability that the diagnosis is mistaken becomes vanishingly small while the condition of the patient in the very rare cases of recovery is one of severe disability, any interest of the patient in continued life-sustaining treatment becomes vanishingly small as well" (Brock 1988, 80). In Brock's defense, at the time of the paper's writing, medical consensus was that the possibility of recovering consciousness after several months in the PVS was vanishingly small.

for patients—Robert Wendland's family, M's partner and family—who can no longer speak for themselves.

6.3.3 Justice

Justice as a bioethical principle is frequently and narrowly framed as concerned primarily with distributive justice and the just allocation and use of limited medical resources. In the context of DoCs, it is sometimes argued that it is unjust to use medical resources to keep alive DoC patients, resources that might be better used to help those who are conscious and who have hope of recovery, or that it would be just to use healthcare monies in some other way that might be more beneficial to society. A crude form of this argument was made by Jacob Appel, who concluded that physicians and hospitals should withhold care from VS patients because it is costly and diverts resources from other, more worthwhile patients and endeavors. We ought, he argued, declare "that the lives of PVS [persistent vegetative state] patients are worth less than those of others."

Money spent on vegetative patients is money not spent on preventive care, such as flu shots and mammograms. Each night in an ICU bed for such patients is a night that another patient with a genuine prognosis for recovery is denied such high-end care. Every dollar exhausted on patients who will never wake up again is a dollar not devoted to finding a cure for cancer. While the *visible* victims may draw the headlines and attract indignant protests from so-called "pro-life" organizations, the *invisible* victims are people like you and me who will suffer from diseases that are never cured because funds are being poured down a healthcare sieve in order to maintain permanently unconscious bodies on complex and costly forms of life support. (2010)[6]

---

[6] Appel was writing about a specific person, Ruben Betancourt, whose family was at the time fighting the hospital that was trying to withdraw LST against their wishes

Aside from the hyperbolic claims about the expense of maintaining VS/UWS patients in ICU beds, the conclusion that healthcare is a zero-sum game (more for one means less for another), or that there is some straightforward financial benefit to denying treatment to DoC patients, is simplistic and naïve, and it pretends that solving the problem of high healthcare costs is as simple as shifting money from column A to column B on some imaginary national medical spreadsheet, resulting in a net benefit (Johnson 2010). It also ignores the very real and substantial social and personal costs of declaring an entire class of patients to be "worth less" and taking away the decisional authority and autonomy of their surrogates and family members.

More sophisticated views of what is required as a matter of distributive justice are less blunt and focus less on the "worth" of these patients, but they can arrive at similar conclusions regarding the allocation of money and medical resources. Brock argued that the aims of medicine cannot be achieved for the PVS patient, and that treatment is effectively futile:

> The promotion of opportunity through the prevention of treatment or treatment of disability is no longer possible since disability is irreversible and total; opportunity presupposes capacities for agency and action. The prevention or palliation of pain and suffering is no longer possible because the capacity for pain and suffering presupposes the consciousness that has been irreversibly lost. (1988, 79)

For Brock, just distributions of healthcare are those that promote opportunity, relieve suffering, and prolong life. He argued that none of these goals can be advanced by providing LST to PVS patients.

(Johnson 2010). Mr. Betancourt was diagnosed in a VS following a medical error during which he was accidentally extubated. He was indeed in the ICU, and receiving expensive medical care, although that is not the norm for chronic VS/UWS patients, who frequently require only basic nursing care and tube feeding.

While such patients may be alive, they derive no benefits from life and have no interest in further life.

Dominic Wilkinson and Julian Savulescu concluded that the economic and welfare burdens of treatment outweigh the welfare benefits for both VS/UWS and MCS patients, and that the benefits of expenditures would be greater if used elsewhere:

> Distributive justice is perhaps the most straightforward ground for limitation of life prolonging treatment since it does not require an answer to the question of whether a person's life is overall worth living, but only an answer to a relative question of whether one life is more worth living or less expensive to support than another. . . . Even if it is of some benefit to be kept alive in an MCS (though we are sceptical of whether the benefits do outweigh the burdens), the magnitude of that benefit is small compared with other uses of limited health resources. (2013, 557–558).

Adopting this kind of Utilitarian calculus might indeed lead to the conclusion that the optimal distribution of healthcare resources—the one that maximizes utility—will be the one that favors those who will benefit more, where the very possibility of benefit and having interests depends on sentience and consciousness. The scales will be tipped toward those with greater capacities for enjoying the benefits, including capacities to enjoy higher-quality, more sophisticated benefits. As John Stuart Mill famously opined,

> It is better to be a human being dissatisfied than a pig satisfied; better to be Socrates dissatisfied than a fool satisfied. And if the fool, or the pig, are of a different opinion, it is because they only know their own side of the question. (1861, 14)

The calculation problem—the difficulty of accurately or even adequately calculating the benefits and burdens of any course of action—has always, and will always, bedevil the Utilitarian calculator. Mill, in rejecting Bentham's supposedly quantifiable and objective felicific calculus, which considered only pleasures and pains, made the calculus immeasurably more complex by demanding that the quality of pleasures and pains be calculated as well. One might think it was made complex to the point of uselessness, and one would have a point. But there's also no Utilitarian reason, in principle, why the simple pleasures (or pains) of an MCS patient should count for less than the sophisticated pleasures of Socrates, or a philosopher, or a neurologist. Perhaps Socrates, or the philosopher, or the neurologist would find it disagreeable to contemplate a future life of only simple pleasures and pains. Perhaps the quality of that life would fall below expectations, to the point that such a life would be, for them, tragic and pointless. So let us add that to the calculus, but individualized for each patient, rather than assigning a value to an entire class of patients. Arriving at ethical judgments and making non-individualized treatment decisions for classes of patients is a nonstarter if justice—even an impoverished view limited to distributive justice—is the goal. Epistemic uncertainties multiply when we attempt to calculate the net benefits of resource distributions across diagnostic categories of patients, not least because the categories themselves are arbitrary, with fuzzy boundaries.

Justice requires that we consider not just individuals and their interests, of course, but also the interests of affected others. A solipsistic or egocentric approach to justice would be nonsensical. In the *Belmont Report*, one of the formative documents on research ethics, the Belmont Commission stated that justice requires that the selection of research subjects

> be scrutinized in order to determine whether some classes (e.g., welfare patients, particular racial and ethnic minorities, or persons confined to institutions) are being systematically selected simply because of their easy availability, their compromised

position, or their manipulability, rather than for reasons directly related to the problem being studied. (1978)

Translated for our purposes here, the vulnerability and disadvantages of marginalized persons should not be exploited to benefit others. In the context of healthcare provision rather than research, justice also demands that the vulnerable and marginalized not be targeted for rationing or cost-cutting, and that they not be excluded from the benefits of medical treatment just because they are easy targets, voiceless, or without societal support, or because they are not valued. This can be clearly applied in the context of DoC patients, where it has frequently been argued that it serves no good purpose to expend resources on individuals—or a class of individuals—who will not benefit or who cannot themselves appreciate the benefits. Note here how this echoes the language of "potentially inappropriate treatment" and patients for whom there is "no reasonable expectation that the patient's neurologic function will improve sufficiently to allow the patient to perceive the benefits of treatment" (Kon et al. 2016).

In times of scarcity and emergency, when crisis standards of care must be invoked—such as during the SARS-CoV-2 pandemic—distribution and allocation issues come to the fore. But as Michael Hickson's story illustrates, patients with brain injuries encounter unjustified preconceptions and biases in healthcare during ordinary times, and those biases, if they in turn inform crisis standards of care, can result in those who are already disabled, vulnerable, or disadvantaged being disadvantaged to death. By necessity, the allocation of a scarce resource during a crisis will be unequal. One goal of allocation decisions is to make what is unequal more equitable. But allocation choices using criteria like the presence of chronic health conditions and disabilities as predictors of survivability reinforce existing structural injustices that disadvantage and burden the poor, the disabled, and persons of color (Johnson 2020a) and exploit preexisting injustices that extend beyond the realm of healthcare—the so-called social determinants of health. Deciding on just allocations of scarce medical resources requires disentangling the thicket of structural and social injustice, discrimination, disease, and disability. Denying a ventilator to a patient with pneumonia because their background health status includes a disability that makes them less likely to survive creates self-fulfilling prophecies that add a veneer of certainty to uncertainty. Denying a ventilator because the patient's quality of life is perceived to be poor or will not be "improved" by a ventilator is in effect saying that the patient's quality of life will not be made worse by dying. And that is another way of saying that the patient's life is not worth living, and not worth saving.

The almost exclusive focus on distributive justice is a symptom of a too narrow view of what justice in healthcare is about and what it requires. While distributive questions demand answers, sometimes urgently, we have not entirely discharged our justice obligations if our answers only maximize utility by calculating the number of lives saved, or years of life saved, or QALYs.[7] Obligations of justice within healthcare require us to think about how healthcare can make society more just, more equitable, more fair, rather than how healthcare can be allocated (or denied) within already unjust societal structures. Working

---

[7] QALYs are quality-adjusted life years, a measurement of cost-effectiveness in health and medicine intended to assist decision-making at multiple levels: the individual clinical level, the programmatic or societal level, and insurance decisions. It uses a preference or desirability scale of 0–1, with 0 being dead and 1 being a state of "perfect" health. Negative values are possible for states worse than death. The preference rating is multiplied by the number of years spent in that state. The purpose is to quantify the value of health-promoting measures based on their contribution to years of life adjusted by quality of life (Weinstein, Torrance, and McGuire 2009). A criticism of QALY is that it is inherently discriminatory against disabled people because health states associated with disability are always rated less than 1, with the result being that prolonging life for someone with a disability is less valuable—less cost-effective—than prolonging life for someone without a disability. VS/UWS is sometimes judged to be a life worse than death and would have a negative QALY rating. Thus, more time in a VS/UWS would be worse than less time, and life-prolonging measures for VS/UWS would not be cost-effective or worth pursuing. It's clear how this kind of calculation informs views like those expressed by Appel, Savulescu, Wilkinson, and Brock above.

out what that means and how it is done are beyond the scope of my project here. But the distributive project of dividing people and patients into classes of gets and get-nots on the basis of diagnosis, or on luck in the genetic/disease/injury/disability lottery, views healthcare as a distributive scalpel for cutting out the unwanted, the disordered, the different. It is incompatible with viewing healthcare as an instrument of justice, of equity, of freedom, of opportunity, and of right treatment, as a corrective not only for what ails us as individuals, but for what ails society, and for how society ails us.

6.3.4 Epistemic Duties

> Though we cannot hinder our knowledge where the agreement is once perceived, nor our assent, where the probability manifestly appears upon due consideration of all the measures of it; yet we can hinder both knowledge and assent, by stopping our inquiry, and not employing our faculties in the search of any truth. If it were not so, ignorance, error, or infidelity, could not in any case be a fault.
>
> This at least is certain, that he must be accountable for whatever mistakes he runs into: whereas he that makes use of the light and faculties God has given him, and seeks sincerely to discover truth, by those helps and abilities he has, may have this satisfaction in doing his duty as a rational creature, that though he should miss truth, he will not miss the reward of it. For he governs his assent right, and places it as he should, who in any case or matter whatsoever, believes or disbelieves, according as reason directs him. He that does otherwise, transgresses against his own light, and misuses those faculties, which were given him. (Locke 1689)

Locke makes two important points here about the epistemic goal of believing all and only truths. The first is that we are blameworthy if we fail to seek knowledge and truth—if we prematurely stop our inquiry. The second is that we are also blameworthy for failing to use our rational faculties—and doing our duty as rational creatures—when we believe or disbelieve without properly considering the evidence before us, "according as reason directs" us. I think both claims are right. We have epistemic duties, as knowers and epistemic agents, both to consider the evidence before us and to seek further evidence when there is uncertainty.

In "The Will to Believe," William James makes a slightly different point about our epistemic duties (or commandments, if you will):

> *We must know the truth; and we must avoid error*—these are our first and great commandments as would-be knowers; but they are not two ways of stating an identical commandment, they are two separable laws. (2014, 17)

For James, if we disbelieve something that is false, we do right, but that's not the end of it. Not believing something that is false, say that the Earth is flat, does not guarantee that we automatically believe or know what is true. We might believe something else that is false, such as that the Earth is a cube. Nor can we discharge our epistemic duties by believing nothing at all about the Earth. Thus, we have a duty to avoid errors in our beliefs, and a duty to know the truth. I focus here on the epistemic duty *to believe all and only truths*—that would seem to require avoiding false beliefs.

James was responding, in "The Will to Believe," to William K. Clifford, who maintained in "The Ethics of Belief" that "It is wrong always, everywhere, and for anyone, to believe anything upon insufficient evidence" (Clifford 1879). That is a high epistemic bar. James was more permissive about when it is acceptable to form beliefs on the basis of insufficient evidence. He thought that there are times, in fact, when we simply must do so, when there is no compelling evidence one way or the other, and we must nonetheless make a choice regarding a momentous issue, because "doing nothing" is also making a choice. This is not unlike the situation surrogates may find themselves in when they must make decisions on behalf of DoC patients. They may not have enough evidence of prior wishes and preferences; there may not be certainty about the patient's current cognitive or psychological states; there may not be certainty about diagnosis and prognosis. Nonetheless, choices must be made.

But perhaps there is an epistemic duty to do better than believe in the face of uncertainty, a duty to actively seek more evidence for our beliefs. Richard Hall and Charles Johnson have argued that if we accept the epistemic goal *to believe all and only truths*, then we also accept an epistemic duty to do what is required to achieve that goal: "Where there are epistemic goals, there are correlative epistemic duties" (Hall and Johnson 1998). This gives rise to a "subjective diachronic epistemic duty to seek more evidence" that "applies to any proposition that is less than certain on our evidence" (Hall and Johnson 1998).

Now, this again seems like a high bar, and one might well sigh and quote the poet: "Had we but world enough and time."[8] But Hall and Johnson distinguish between epistemic agents who believe propositions that are not objectively certain and those who believe propositions about which they are subjectively uncertain. The former—say, someone who believes in the existence of unicorns—is not epistemically blameworthy if they have no way of knowing they have false or uncertain beliefs. But the latter knower, who

---

[8] From "To His Coy Mistress" by Andrew Marvell (https://www.poetryfoundation.org/poems/44688/to-his-coy-mistress). William P. Alston did quote the poet and concluded, "We could require people to carry out an exhaustive investigation of each witness, search through all the relevant literature for considerations pertinent to each candidate for belief, check each calculation ten times. . . . But we simply do not have time for that" (Alston 1988).

harbors subjective uncertainty about some proposition, is blame-worthy if they fail in their epistemic duty to seek more evidence.

So. Locke maintained that we fail in our duty as rational creatures if we fail to seek knowledge and truth by stopping inquiry, and if we fail to properly consider the evidence before us. Hall and Johnson described an epistemic duty to seek more evidence in the face of known objective and subjective uncertainty. James enjoined us to seek truth and avoid error, but he acknowledged that, practically speaking, there are times when we must make choices in the midst of uncertainty. I think that's all right.

6.3.4.1 Distributive Epistemic Justice

> *Ipsa scientia potestas est. (Knowledge itself is power.)*
> —Francis Bacon in the *Meditationes sacrae* (1597)

We should consider some epistemic agents blameworthy for failing to seek more evidence. Specifically, epistemic agents who are in the right position to know that there is uncertainty about a proposition, and who are in the right position to obtain the evidence that either confirms or relieves that uncertainty, are blameworthy for failing to seek more evidence. More specifi-cally, physicians and other medical staff are the kinds of epistemic agents who are in such a position with respect to the fact of un-certainty concerning diagnosis and prognosis of DoCs. And they are the epistemic agents with access to the evidence of that un-certainty and its implications. Because they endorse the epistemic goal of believing all and only true beliefs within their sphere of ex-pertise (or so one hopes), and they can seek and find the relevant evidence, and indeed, it is within their job description and their professional codes of ethics to be well informed and current in their knowledge, they can, and do, have the epistemic duty to seek more evidence. The evidence, at present, is abundant concerning misdiagnosis and uncertainty about DoCs.

What does it mean, in this context, to seek more evidence? It does not mean that every doctor, every neurologist, or every neurointensivist must shift their career into research on DoCs. It means, simply, that they have an epistemic duty to remain current on the relevant research that is already being done. They need not, contrary to Alston, themselves carry out an exhaustive investigation and check each calculation ten times. The "duty to seek more evidence applies to any proposition that is less than certain on our evidence," and that duty extends to knowing that there is uncertainty. The blameworthy epistemic agent fails to know that there is uncertainty when they should, and could, know that. Uncertainty is a known fact about DoCs, and not knowing it is epistemically irresponsible. The evidence that misdiagnosis has been a serious problem in VS/UWS has been repeatedly affirmed for decades. The belief that a VS/UWS diagnosis is immune to error is false, and it is not based on the available evidence. If diagnosis is uncertain, so is prognosis informed by diagnosis. Denying the fact would be epistemically irresponsible.

Whereas diagnosis of VS/UWS is on average wrong in about 40 percent of cases, that does not translate to a 4 in 10 chance of being wrong about a specific patient. Indeed, depending on the patient, the risks of being wrong might be lower or higher. In other words, there is also uncertainty about the uncertainty at the level of individual patients. Such circumstances call for epistemic humility.

> Epistemic humility does not reject clinical expertise. Rather, epistemic humility encourages [healthcare providers] to consider the limits of clinical expertise, especially where there is uncertainty or incomplete knowledge about a clinical situation. (Buchman, Ho, and Goldberg 2017)

The importance of epistemic humility is amplified by the vulnerability of patients and their surrogates. Regarding complex clinical information, they are frequently at an epistemic disadvantage and dependent on medical staff to provide and help them interpret and contextualize that information. Unlike doctors and other medical staff, they generally lack access to medical journals, and they lack the expertise to understand information produced for professional audiences. And, as Buchman, Ho, and Goldberg pointed out, since medical staff are "gatekeepers of resources and are the ones with the official credentials to treat patients, if they are not trustworthy, patients would be vulnerable to betrayal" (Buchman, Ho, and Goldberg 2017, 32). Thus, patients and surrogates can frequently be in a situation in which they know too little, have too little access to reliable, relevant information, and must trust their doctors. The epistemic asymmetry makes them epistemically vulnerable and dependent on others.

> In trusting healthcare professionals, patients are taking a risk because they assume that their medical insight is inferior to that of the professionals, who will use their knowledge in a beneficial way. Their trust makes them vulnerable and dependent, as the knowledge difference renders it difficult for them to challenge their healthcare professionals' judgements, which forces them to trust the treatment and care offered. Thus, all patient–healthcare professional relationships are more or less asymmetric. This epistemic asymmetry is caused by one party having skills and knowledge that the other party does not have but needs. (Alpers 2018)

Fricker described *distributive epistemic injustice* as "the unfair distribution of epistemic goods such as education or information" (Fricker 2013). That healthcare professionals have access to specialized knowledge is not unfair and is not itself an instance of epistemic injustice. Most professions involve specialized training and distribution of knowledge, where the latter is dependent on the former. But patients and surrogates are vulnerable and must trust healthcare workers because of the epistemic asymmetry of medical knowledge. For that reason, medical staff have additional distributive epistemic duties to them. Thus, we return to the concept of *distributive justice* in healthcare, but here the resource being distributed is knowledge or information.

We can describe it thusly: The epistemic goal of believing all and only true beliefs has the correlative epistemic duty to seek evidence where there is uncertainty. The epistemic goal is shared by patients and surrogates, but they lack the epistemic resources (knowledge, training, access to evidence) to seek evidence or even to know that there is uncertainty. Those who have the knowledge, access, and resources have a duty to share needed information as a matter of justice. Doing so contributes to the epistemic goal of believing all and only true beliefs. Withholding such information impairs the patient's or surrogate's ability to act as an epistemic agent and must therefore count as a form of distributive epistemic injustice.

This idea is contained in the ideal of voluntary informed consent. Individuals have a right to control what happens to their bodies in the context of medical treatment. In order for a patient to provide voluntary informed consent for medical treatment, they must be free of coercion and must have enough information about their treatment options to provide consent that is informed. Withholding information could be coercive—it could direct patients toward options they would not otherwise choose. It would constitute a violation of their autonomy as well, since their consent would not be informed. But it would also exploit the epistemic asymmetry that exists between medical staff, and patients and surrogates. Clearly, informed consent does not require a patient to acquire the same level of knowledge or information that a physician has. A patient need not be able to perform surgery to consent to surgery. But it is just as clear that some information deficiencies or lacunas can hinder meaningful informed consent.

6.3.4.2 Amy Reed and the Duty to Inform

Amy Reed was an anesthesiologist. She had six children with her husband, Hooman Norchashm, a cardiothoracic surgeon. In 2013,

Reed had surgery at Brigham & Women's Hospital in Boston to remove uterine fibroids. She was not told that a power morcellator, a surgical tool that uses a rotating blade to chop up and remove benign fibroids and uterine tissue, would be used in her surgery. Power morcellation allows for less invasive and faster surgeries, with easier recovery for patients, but it has the potential to spread hidden, malignant tumors. A biopsy after her surgery revealed that Reed's fibroids were hiding leiomyosarcoma, an aggressive form of cancer that had been spread throughout her abdominal cavity by the morcellator. By the time she was diagnosed, she had Stage IV cancer and needed several surgeries and radiotherapy to treat metastatic tumors.

As it happened, the same fate had befallen another patient, Erica Kaitz, who had the same surgery at the same hospital, and who died of the same cancer just 3 months after Reed's surgery (Ong 2017). Reed and her husband engaged in a very public campaign against the use of power morcellation for gynecologic surgeries like hers, even as she was dying. She died in May 2017 at the age of 44, 3 years and 7 months after her surgery.

The Food and Drug Administration (FDA) issued its final guidance on the use of power morcellation in December 2020, recognizing the not remote possibility of hidden sarcomas:

> The FDA estimates that a hidden uterine sarcoma may be present in approximately 1 in 225 to 1 in 580 women undergoing surgery for uterine fibroids based on recent publications. The FDA also estimates that a leiomyosarcoma (a specific type of uterine sarcoma) may be present in approximately 1 in 495 to 1 in 1100 women undergoing surgery for uterine fibroids based on recent studies. Prior to 2014, the clinical community estimated uterine sarcomas to be present much less frequently, in as few as 1 in 10,000 women undergoing surgery for uterine fibroids.
>
> Several studies show that using a laparoscopic power morcellator during gynecologic surgery in women with hidden

uterine sarcomas is associated with lowering their chances of long-term survival without cancer. While these studies have limitations, women who have had fibroid surgery with a laparoscopic power morcellator later found to have a hidden uterine sarcoma, have lower disease-free survival (less time without any sign or symptom of cancer after surgery), when compared to women who were treated with manual morcellation or without morcellation. In addition, there is data to suggest an increase in rate of occult sarcoma for women undergoing surgery for presumed fibroids.

Uterine sarcomas and uterine fibroids may have similar signs and symptoms. At this time, there is no reliable method for predicting or testing whether a woman with fibroids may have a uterine sarcoma.

The FDA recommends healthcare providers share this information with patients and warns against using laparoscopic power morcellators in gynecologic surgeries to treat patients with suspected or confirmed cancer, and in women over age 50 having a myomectomy or hysterectomy for uterine fibroids. (2020)

The FDA's statement contains a number of points of interest. It notes the *estimated* rates of hidden sarcomas, and how that estimate changed after Dr. Reed's experience. It notes the uncertainty that exists both in estimating the risk of "disease-free survival" (a tortured euphemism for surviving without metastasis linked to the use of power morcellation), and the inherent uncertainty caused by the lack of a "reliable method for predicting or testing" whether fibroids harbor hidden sarcomas. And it recommends that healthcare providers share this information with their patients.[9]

---

[9] The FDA made several other recommendations for device manufacturers regarding the labeling of their devices, including a warning to healthcare providers that the use of power morcellators is contraindicated in gynecologic surgeries where tissue is known or suspected to contain malignancy. Since there is no way to reliably know which fibroids might contain malignancies, this would seem to rule out any use of power morcellators to remove fibroids.

A "recommendation" to share information is hardly strong enough to describe what is a manifest duty to inform patients of the risks of power morcellation surgery in metastasizing a deadly disease. The risks are relatively small—.17 to .44 percent—but the seriousness of the risks, which include severe illness, onerous treatments, and death, warrants more than a recommendation. Informing patients of such risks should not be optional. We can apply the First Principle of Inductive Risk to the power morcellation story in two instances. The first concerns the use of these devices in gynecologic surgeries. Recall that the tolerable level of epistemic risk is set by the ethical risks of being wrong. The more serious the ethical risks, the lower should be our tolerance for epistemic risk-taking. So, even given the estimated pre-2014 risk of sarcoma in 1 in 10,000 women undergoing surgery, the ethical seriousness of the risk—severe illness and death—argues against the use of power morcellation as unacceptably risky. The First Principle of Inductive Risk tells us that our epistemic standard—our level of epistemic certainty about safety—should be quite high when it comes to using power morcellation in gynecologic surgeries, because the ethical risks are quite high. In addition, even though the estimated risk of sarcoma was low (1 in 10,000), there existed uncertainty because there was no reliable way to know which fibroids would be malignant until after the fact (and in fact, the risk is now estimated to be 44 times higher). Thus, there was also an epistemic duty to seek more evidence of safety.

The second application of the principle is relevant now as well, when the risks associated with power morcellation are known to be much higher. The inductive risks still argue against the use of power morcellation. The uncertainty about which fibroids will hide deadly sarcomas requires that epistemic agents (in this case, gynecologists and gynecologic surgeons) seek more evidence, know the fact (or truth, as James might say) of uncertainty, and importantly, enable other epistemic agents, their patients, to know about the uncertainty by informing them. This is not optional, and warning patients of these risks is not supererogatory. It is an epistemic duty to inform.

Now consider the risks of misdiagnosis in DoC. About 40 percent of patients diagnosed in the VS/UWS—patients diagnosed as unconscious—are misdiagnosed. They are conscious and aware. They might be minimally conscious, with possible capacities for experiencing pain and positive and negative psychological states. They might be more than minimally conscious, with CMD, which includes a range of cognitive capacities. The epistemic risk there is significantly higher (about 20 times higher) than in the power morcellation case. The risks of being wrong have less to do with the skill or experience of the physician performing an assessment and more to do with the tests, the mismatch between the tests and what they test for, and the inherent inaccessibility of another's inner cognitive states.

But in the case of DoCs, the risks are not so much in the diagnosis itself, but in what is done with that information. And what is done with that information includes making judgments about the value of life for that patient and what that patient would want, as well as making decisions about continuing and discontinuing LST. There is a risk that surrogates and others participating in decision-making on behalf of DoC patients will not be adequately informed of the epistemic uncertainty of DoCs and will make decisions— because they must, always—based on beliefs they acquire with insufficient evidence. That is, they will be thwarted in achieving the shared epistemic goal of believing all and only truths. They will be thwarted not because information is nonexistent, but because they do not have the epistemic resources to acquire the information that exists. And so, gatekeeper epistemic agents with access to knowledge of the uncertainty (i.e., medical staff) have a duty to inform other epistemic agents (i.e., patient surrogates) of the uncertainty. Their failure to do so maintains epistemic asymmetries, maintains ignorance by withholding available epistemic resources, and impedes disadvantaged epistemic agents from acquiring needed information.

This failure might be attributed to epistemic paternalism, in which information is withheld from an agent, without their consent, for their own *epistemic* good (to avoid misunderstandings or confusion, perhaps, or to avoid overwhelming an epistemic agent with too much information), or to an epistemic nudge, in which information is presented in a certain way (after all, it unavoidably must be presented in some way) to facilitate people choosing in the ways that are best for them. But it might also be an instance of epistemic *manipulation*, in which some facts are intentionally left out or not presented for non-epistemic reasons (Jackson 2021), such as doing what is in the interests of a hospital or society. It may be some combination of these, but regardless of the motive or justification, they all count as some kind of epistemic *interference* in that they impede or interfere with an epistemic agent's achievement of their epistemic goals, and with their right to know.

David Coady has argued that a person can have their right to know something violated in two distinct ways:

> They can be unjustly put (or left) in a position in which they are ignorant of something that they are entitled to know, or they can be unjustly put (or left) in a position in which they are wrong about something they are entitled to be right about. There seems no reason to think that either of these is inherently more of an injustice than the other. (2010, 109)

Thus, another form of epistemic injustice is what Coady describes as "unjust ignorance or error" (Coady 2010, 110), and it is both a moral and an epistemic kind of injustice. It is related to *distributive epistemic injustice*, or an unjust distribution (or nondistribution) of knowledge or information. What makes it unjust, as Coady noted, is that it constitutes a violation of someone's right to know, or their right not to be left believing in error. It's an epistemic injustice in that it thwarts an epistemic agent's goal of believing true beliefs, and it's a moral injustice because true beliefs have instrumental moral value. In the context of DoCs, having true beliefs about the diagnosis and prognosis for the person you are making decisions for is vitally important.

6.3.4.3 Antidotes to Injustice

The antidote to this injustice, if it is motivated by epistemic paternalism (or nudging), by a desire to achieve what is best for an epistemic agent, is epistemic humility. Epistemic humility requires acknowledging the limits of one's own knowledge, including knowledge about what is in someone else's interests. As noted above, it is not necessarily a deficiency in the skills or knowledge of a physician that is at the root of errors in diagnosis and prognosis in the context of DoCs. Thus, epistemic humility also requires acknowledging the limits of the body of knowledge in one's profession or specialty (e.g., that there is a high rate of misdiagnosis of the VS/UWS; that there is no reliable way to know if uterine fibroids are cancerous). Transparency is how epistemic humility is applied and transmitted to other epistemic agents who have the need and the right to know.

Epistemic *manipulation* calls for a different remedy: the assertion of the rights of patients and surrogates against manipulation and exploitation. As discussed above, when the concept of justice in healthcare is limited to distributive justice, brain-injured and DoC patients are vulnerable to exploitation of their marginalization through the distributive project of using healthcare as a scalpel to cut out the unwanted, the disordered, and the different. Viewing epistemic manipulation as a violation of *epistemic rights* and a matter of *epistemic distributive justice* allows us to see how medical knowledge empowers, and how withholding it disempowers and exploits unjust ignorance. Thus, epistemic manipulation is unjust in all the ways that other forms of manipulation in medicine and healthcare are unjust. For the same reasons that manipulation and exploitation are unethical in non-epistemic medical contexts, they are unethical in the distribution of knowledge and information to patients and their surrogates. Withholding knowledge and information is a violation of the professional duties of medical staff, and a violation of their duties as epistemic agents.

It is not possible to make decisions if we are paralyzed by uncertainty. As James said, there are times when we simply must make choices and decisions without having conclusive evidence one way or another, and indeed we can have moral obligations to do so. Those moral duties may well take precedence over epistemic duties at times. But because ethically important and risky decisions and choices must be made under conditions of uncertainty, some epistemic agents have a *moral* duty to fulfill their epistemic duties. That is why the specific failure of medical staff as epistemic agents to know and *acknowledge* uncertainty, and to practice epistemic humility, is a matter of epistemic justice, and an ethical failure as well. It fails to respect the autonomy of patients and their surrogates, it fails to act with beneficence and nonmaleficence, and it fails to advance justice.

6.4 The Ethics of Uncertainty

Let's take stock and consider DoCs as our case study for what I call the ethics of uncertainty.

We face ineluctable, entangled uncertainties. Epistemic and ontological uncertainty about consciousness and its absence. Epistemic uncertainty about inferences and about how much ethical weight they can bear, and uncertainty because of the necessity of inferences in the presence of epistemic lacunas. Uncertainty about DoCs, about what they are, and about their proper boundaries. Uncertainty about DoC patients, and their proper categories, about what they experience and don't, about what they think or don't think, about what they can do or know, and about their interests, if they have any. Ethical uncertainties about what is best, about what rights and interests have priority, about who lives and who dies, and how they live and die, and about how to decide and who decides. And again, the entangled uncertainties here—the ontological, epistemic, and ethical—are such that, even if we reduce or eliminate uncertainty in one realm, we will still be left with uncertainties in the others.

I have expressed skepticism about the possibility of universal moral conclusions and prescriptions given all this uncertainty. Even if we accept that such prescriptions are possible in theory, there are reasons to doubt that we could adequately apply them under conditions of uncertainty such as exist concerning DoCs, and other circumstances with comparable uncertainty. One fact about ethical prescriptions concerning DoCs and DoC patients is the long-standing tendency to conclude that questions about what should be done *for* or *about* all DoC patients can be answered with certainty by considering the importance and value of consciousness and unconsciousness, without attending to the uncertainty of consciousness and unconsciousness.

Concerning some principled prescriptions common to bioethics—to respect autonomy, to act beneficently and nonmaleficently, to act justly—we have seen that the same reasons that exist generally also apply in the case of DoCs, although the uncertainties vex our efforts, as they did for those deciding on behalf of Robert Wendland and M. I've also offered two other principles that index uncertainty to epistemic and ethical risk-taking, which I call the First and Second Principles of Inductive Risk. I take these principles to contribute less to making actions and decisions right rather than wrong than to cultivating moral decision-making that is better under the epistemic circumstances. The principles contribute to actions and decisions that are more likely to consider moral reasons, and more likely to counteract biases, misconceptions, faulty evidence, and error. They are principles that can help us be better epistemic and moral agents.

Finally, I argued that we must consider justice and its demands, in the face of uncertainty, far more expansively than has typically been done when thinking about DoCs. The almost exclusive focus on where DoC patients fit in the allocation of medical resources has led many to rest their case on the supposed fact of unconsciousness, and to conclude that the lives of the unconscious are of so little value—to themselves or to others—that they are simply not worth the candle. But there is more to justice than totting up costs and benefits on an imaginary spreadsheet. Here again, the epistemic uncertainties bubble up to the surface, and reveal the distinctly *epistemic* duties and injustices that demand action. Those injustices are also distributive in nature, but they concern the distribution of knowledge and information. Medical staff have epistemic duties to acknowledge the uncertainty and to seek evidence about DoCs. They have a duty to inform patient surrogates—who share the epistemic goal of believing all and only truths about DoCs and about the patient they must decide for—about the uncertainties, because surrogates are at an epistemic disadvantage and are vulnerable.

Medical staff, as trusted epistemic agents with access to knowledge and information, have a duty to remedy epistemic asymmetries, epistemic paternalism, manipulation, and exploitation, and to act with epistemic humility, as a matter of respecting rights, and as a matter of justice. Their epistemic duties include indexing the inductive and ethical risks and uncertainties required to address the Problem of Inductive Risk in DoCs: given ethical risks, what is the appropriate epistemic standard of evidence for accepting a diagnosis? The First Principle of Inductive Risk tells us to index epistemic risk-taking to the ethical risks of being wrong. The greater the ethical risks of being wrong, the less epistemic risk we should tolerate. Applying this principle requires epistemic humility. It requires acknowledging the limits of knowledge, the very real risk of diagnostic error in DoCs, and the related prognostic risks. The Second Principle of Inductive Risk tells us to index ethical risk-taking to the epistemic risks of being wrong. There, the greater the epistemic uncertainty, the less tolerance we should have for ethical risk-taking. The second principle places a heavy burden on surrogates. They must find a balance between the epistemic uncertainty and the very real, very specific ethical risks that will exist as a result of their choices, and perform a complex calculation involving numerous variables (some of them also of uncertain value).

The ethics of uncertainty is sensitive and responsive to epistemic uncertainty that comes with ethical risks, and to where epistemic and ethical uncertainty interact. These conditions are not exclusive to decision-making concerning DoC patients. Indeed, because uncertainty is so common in medical contexts, it adapts readily to the problems encountered in other areas of healthcare. Like all applications of ethics worth their salt, the ethics of uncertainty requires attention to rights, and to beneficence and nonmaleficence. Always and everywhere, we are obligated to respect the rights of persons, and try to help, and not harm. The ethics of uncertainty also requires an expansive view of the demands of justice that importantly—necessarily—includes epistemic justice. Epistemic justice and the duties of epistemic agents are, as I have described them, quite demanding.

6.5 Disorders of Consciousness and All Things Considered

Consider again the matter of withdrawing LST in acute neurointensive care. The problem I identified there is twofold. There is an epistemic problem: an unacceptable degree of uncertainty about prognosis, and the potential for actions to lead to self-fulfilling prophecies. There is an ethical problem: real and significant ethical risks that include premature death when life would have been preferable, and continued life when death would have been preferable. Actions and decisions with ethically important consequences in the context of acute care after brain injuries can thus be better or worse, all things considered. Considering *all things* includes considering contextual features that are specific to individuals, their surrogates, their families, their resources, their cultures and communities, and facts about their societies and the level and kinds of societal support and resources available. Importantly, when treatment decisions are made for patients, they are always made under non-ideal conditions, and facts about those non-ideal conditions and the ways that they are non-ideal, also count in moral reasoning when making choices with ethical implications and consequences.

Our goal ought not be to hold the decisions of surrogates to the standard of clean, consistent, abstract, ideal decision-making in an ideal world. Our goal ought not be consistency for its own sake—for example, to always withdraw treatment or always continue treatment when a patient is diagnosed with a devastating brain injury or in a VS/UWS. Nor should we maintain that some principle—say, the sanctity of life—can always override other considerations or serve as a tiebreaker (as it might have done in M's case). In the real, non-ideal world, things get messy and complicated, emotional, needful, and rife with conflicts. Demanding consistency or holding fast to absolute principles might well be cruel. We ought to avoid cruelty and avoid making hard choices even harder.

The approach to decision-making and acting that is appropriate in the context of uncertainty and DoCs (or other brain injuries) is what I elsewhere call the *All Things Considered* approach.[10] It acknowledges the very real choice constraints that decision makers face. The relevant features of decisions and decision-making for DoC patients are varied and massively contextual in a way that challenges theoretical or principled approaches and prescriptions. Some of the features are *uncertain* and profoundly specific to the person, including diagnosis and prognosis, the potential for

---

[10] See Johnson and Cerminara (2020) for details on what this approach can look like in action.

recovery, the extent or level of recovery (although these can be, in some cases and to some extent, dependent on the treatment and rehabilitative services available). These fierce uncertainties are magnified by the need to consider the patient's preferences, values, and beliefs. While those values and preferences may be clear and unequivocal for some patients or in some situations (for example, the elderly patient with an absolute, unambiguous, standing Do Not Resuscitate/Do Not Intubate order), they are more frequently ambiguous and require much interpretation in the unruly situations surrogates actually face when deciding for DoC patients with unpredictable, uncertain futures. Sometimes there is little to no information about what the patient would want (for example, if the patient is a child, or an adult who never had the capacity to formulate or express their preferences, like Sheila Pouliot). And in some cultures, it is the norm for such decisions to be wholly left to family members, although that does not mean they can or do act without considering what the patient would want, or what is best for them under the circumstances. Some of the features are *certain* but specific to a time and place, including financial and societal resource constraints over which individuals have little control, such as how well one's health insurance covers rehabilitation, long-term nursing care, or home-based care, and what level and kind of societal resources are available that could affect treatment and rehabilitation, accommodations, opportunities, and inclusion in work and school.

But so it goes. Life and death questions are complicated. The point that bears emphasizing (again) is that these questions, as they concern patients with brain injuries and DoCs, are very, very complicated and specific to individuals—more so than has often been recognized and acknowledged.

PART III
SOME APPLICATIONS

7

Moral Status and
the Consciousness Criterion

Moral status and *person* and *personhood* are sometimes used to mean
the same thing: mattering morally. Sometimes *person* is used to designate someone with the highest, or most, moral status, suggesting
that there are different levels of moral status that different entities, or a
single entity at different times, might have. An entity with moral status
is *someone*, not some *thing*. It matters, in a moral sense, what others
do to, and for, them. The use of *person* and *moral status* interchangeably is tendentious, perhaps invidious, because in common parlance,
person is frequently taken to mean all and only humans. I am going
to refer to humans with moral status as *persons*. I am mostly speaking
of humans in this chapter, so this usage will not strike most readers
as odd. (I don't think there is anything odd about calling nonhuman
animals with moral status persons where *person* just picks out their
moral status.)[1]

Some persons are not moral agents—they lack some or all
of the capacities needed to be moral agents.[2] Those capacities

---

[1] I extend my thanks to Nada Gligorov and the attendees of the Working Papers in
Ethics and Moral Psychology meeting (November 19, 2020, via pandemic Zoom) and to
my colleagues in the Center for Bioethics and Humanities, who heard earlier, more rambling versions of this chapter as a work-in-progress. That it is less rambling than it once
was is no doubt due to their helpful and thoughtful comments.

[2] There may be degrees of moral agency. For example, there is compelling evidence
that some nonhuman animals, such as dogs and nonhuman primates, demonstrate
moral agency—they regulate their own behavior in accordance with the demands of justice and altruism. Similarly, very young children demonstrate sensitivity to moral principles like justice and fairness, even if they lack the capacities to engage in sophisticated
reasoning about such principles. On a traditional, strict view of moral agency, it requires
sophisticated reasoning, autonomy, and free will, and behaving in moral ways for moral

include being able to self-regulate their behavior in response to the demands of morality. Moral agents act (or reason) according to moral principles, act (or reason) altruistically, or justly, or fairly, and can recognize and respect the rights of others. Being a moral agent requires, minimally, being autonomous and capable of reasoning. Persons who are not moral agents are moral subjects or moral patients to whom moral agents have duties and obligations. They also matter morally.

The term *person* also has legal meaning, in which it picks out entities who are the subjects of legal rights. Thus, we might think one could be a person morally speaking and not be a legal person. That is, one could be a moral agent or moral subject, someone to whom *moral* consideration is due, and not be a legal person. We might think, for example, that chimpanzees or Thor or Murderbot or Frankenstein's monster or angels are persons—they are due moral consideration—but they are not legally recognized as persons here on Earth, where only humans are legally recognized as persons (whereas humans might not be legal "persons" on some other world, or on a future Earth ruled by intelligent apes).

In the philosophical and bioethical discourses on disorders of consciousness (DoCs), *moral status*, *person*, and *human* are not always treated as synonymous. That is, not all humans are thought to be persons. Some humans—such as those with chronic impairments of consciousness—are sometimes thought to have limited moral status and so are not regarded as persons, and thus don't matter as much as persons do. This prompts some to propose convoluted and arbitrary criteria and justifications for who is, and who is not, a person. I'm a pluralist about persons and personhood, and about mattering morally. I think there are many entities who

reasons. Mark Rowlands has argued that human and nonhuman animals who *act for moral reasons*, even if they cannot reflect on those reasons, are moral subjects (Rowlands 2012). David DeGrazia has maintained that "there are different kinds and degrees of moral agency, and that the crude statement that no nonhuman animals are moral agents cannot be sustained" (DeGrazia 1996, 204).

are persons, and many ways to be a person. In other words, many entities (including, but not only, humans) have moral status.

In this chapter, my aim is not to provide a positive account of moral status and personhood. Rather, my aim is to show why consciousness is not a suitable criterion for determining who is, and who is not, a person with moral status. I am skeptical that there are defensible, necessary, nonmoral criteria for a moral property like "personhood" or "moral status." But assuming there are such criteria, they would need to meet a high standard of epistemic certainty given the inductive risks. Consciousness would fail to satisfy the demands of epistemic certainty, especially in the hard cases involving DoCs. So, I argue here that there are at least three reasons to reject the Consciousness Criterion: the irreducibility of moral personhood to a nonmoral property like consciousness; that there are no defensible necessary criteria for personhood; and the epistemic uncertainty of consciousness and the problem of inductive risk.

7.1 The Consciousness Criterion

The idea that consciousness imbues an entity with special value, or moral status, is widely accepted in Western cultures. As Valerie Hardcastle described it,

> Many people (perhaps most people) believe that being conscious elevates one's moral status in the world. . . . This is, in fact, a deeply held premise in most folks' moral reasoning—so deep, in fact, that we do not bother to defend that premise in moral discussions, science policy briefs, or medical texts. Indeed, we rarely even acknowledge its existence. (2016, 211)

The Consciousness Criterion is the claim that moral status requires consciousness, or that being conscious is a necessary condition for being a person. For now, I'll set aside any questions about whether personhood is exclusive to humans and consider the moral status of typically functioning adult humans (TFAHs) as the status of being persons. *Typically functioning* includes having a capacity for consciousness. As an ethical claim, the Consciousness Criterion has been applied to DoCs (and brain death) from the start, but it has had a long life as a metaphysical claim as well. In some more nuanced versions of the claim, a particular type or level of consciousness is necessary for personhood.

The Consciousness Criterion involves at least one of two claims:

1. Personhood requires consciousness. Call this the *General Consciousness Criterion.*
2. Personhood requires a particular type of consciousness. Call this the *Particular Consciousness Criterion.*

Suppose, as is commonly done, that there is a presumptive moral status—personhood—that TFAHs have by virtue of X. That presumptive status gives them a presumptive moral right against being harmed, which includes a claim to resources like life-sustaining treatment (or, more generally, a right to life). We can state this concisely by saying that *typically functioning adult humans are persons with rights, including a defeasible right to life.* Without X, they do not have that moral status, they are not persons, and they have no claim to the resources needed to keep them alive. Versions of these claims have also been deployed in abortion arguments concerning the moral status or personhood of fetuses.[3] Moral status and criteria for personhood are also commonly invoked in animal ethics/animal

---

[3] Abortion and DoCs dominate the bioethical discourse on personhood. There is a spectrum of views on the personhood of fetuses/embryos. John Noonan, for example, argued that conception by human parents, or genetic humanity, is the definitive condition (Noonan 1970). At the other end of the spectrum, Michael Tooley, echoing Locke, proposed that a person must have particular types of mental states, specifically "a concept of a self as a continuing subject of experiences and other mental states" (Tooley 1972). Mary Anne Warren set the bar similarly high with a set of five criteria that include consciousness, reasoning, communication, and self-awareness (Warren 1973). These latter two positions are both consistent with the Consciousness Criterion. Both Tooley

rights discourse. Humans with contested moral status (or question-able personhood, as it were) are so-called *marginal cases*. Marginal cases involve entities that are like TFAHs in some ways and different from TFAHs in other ways. The question concerning marginal cases is whether they possess X—the relevant properties or characteristics that ground moral status/personhood.[4] Depending on what we think X is, an entity can have always had X, can acquire X, or can lose X, and correspondingly have, acquire, or lose personhood.

In the context of DoCs, only the consciousness and moral status of humans are under consideration, so we can set aside considerations of other entities for the time being. On the General Consciousness Criterion view, X is consciousness, and conscious humans are persons. To be human but unconscious is to no longer be a person. So, it is *consciousness* and not humanity doing the moral work in the case of the unconscious human, since human - consciousness $\neq$ person. Similarly for the Particular Consciousness Criterion view, X is a specific conscious capacity (sentience, phenomenal consciousness, access consciousness, self-awareness). That specific type of

and Warren acknowledged that their criteria were compatible with denying personhood and a right to live to infants. Tooley accepted that infanticide was morally permissible, while Warren claimed infanticide was impermissible because other persons would object to the killing of an infant. Baruch Brody took a somewhat intermediate position, that it is the onset of "encephalographic activity" that matters (Brody 1982), and considered it an advantage of his view that encephalographic activity is measurable and can be used to determine both the beginning and the end of personhood. Presumably, Tooley's and Warren's criteria can be similarly deployed to determine the end of personhood. Indeed, that is essentially how the Consciousness Criterion functions in bioethical discussions of DoCs—the loss of consciousness entails the loss of personhood.

[4] What is referred to as the *problem of marginal cases* is this: if we bootstrap nontypically functioning humans (infants, persons with severe cognitive/intellectual disabilities, etc.) into the moral status club, moral consistency demands that we should either include nonhuman animals who have capacities similar (or superior) to, say, a human infant, or show that there are morally relevant, consistent (nonspeciesist) reasons for excluding them. In the animal ethics literature, the argument from marginal cases is sometimes referred to as the argument from species overlap (Horta 2014) because it rests on the overlapping capacities of the cases in question. What the argument specifically rules out is using species membership (e.g., being human) to decide who matters morally. In environmental ethics, the debate extends to the grounds for the moral status or moral considerability of human, animal, and nonanimal entities, such as trees, lakes, and ecosystems (Hale 2011).

consciousness matters morally. On both views, consciousness is a necessary condition for moral status or personhood. Now, if moral status admits of degrees, then it's possible that some humans are persons (with full moral status) and some have some other moral status between being a person and being a mere thing, depending on whether they manifest the right kind of consciousness.

Arguments about the moral status and ethics of marginal cases typically begin by making claims about the *nonmoral* properties or capacities an entity possesses. From there, conclusions are drawn about the *moral* properties that entity does or does not have, such as a right to life, liberty rights, a right not to be harmed, moral agency, personhood, and so on. The general idea is that moral status reduces to possession of certain moral or nonmoral properties. This line of argument implies, again, that there can be more than one possible status, more than one degree of mattering morally. It's also possible to have no moral status at all. One could assume, for example, that a chair, although replete with nonmoral properties (soft, well-worn, cat-scratched) has no moral properties and thus no moral status. A chair is not the sort of thing that is a candidate for some sort of moral status. But marginal cases *might* be. What are the nonmoral properties that might make one the sort of entity that has moral status? After all, a human might also be soft, well-worn, and cat-scratched, but, presumably, those are not the sort of properties that bear on whether or not a human has moral status.

Our question is whether consciousness is the right sort of property to be X.

7.2 Metaphysical Personhood, Moral Agency, and Consciousness

In modern philosophical discourse on personhood, the connection between personhood and consciousness has roots in the

Lockean idea that a person is "a thinking intelligent Being, that has reason and reflection, and can consider itself as itself, the same thinking thing in different times and places" (Locke 1689). Locke also identified diachronic psychological identity of persons with self-consciousness:

> In this alone consists *personal Identity*, i.e. the sameness of rational Being: And as far as this consciousness can be extended backwards to any past Action or Thought, so far reaches the Identity of that *Person*; it is the same *self* now it was then; and 'tis by the same *self* with this present one that now reflects on it, that that Action was done. (1689)

Locke here asserted that the intelligence, rationality, and capacity to think of themselves persisting over time makes persons capable of anticipating punishments and rewards connected to their actions. That is, persons with diachronic self-consciousness can be moral agents. In contemporary bioethical discourses, Locke's ontology has been stretched into a moral prescription about what (or who) matters.

7.2.1 The General Consciousness Criterion

As discussed in chapter 2, the idea that unconscious humans are no longer persons took hold in both the public imagination and the philosophical and bioethical discourses as soon as the PVS was named and described. Fletcher, in "Four Indicators of Humanhood," considered "what is a *person*" and identified as the cardinal "hominizing" trait "neocortical function" (Fletcher 1974). Fletcher conflated humanity and personhood, with the unfortunate result that when he denied the personhood of some entity, he also denied their humanity (literally, he denied their species membership), as part of his effort to link personhood to biology.

Neocortical function is the key to humanness, the essential trait, the human sine qua non. . . . Without the synthesizing function of the cerebral cortex (without thought or mind), whether before it is present or with its end, the person is nonexistent no matter how much the individual's brain stem and mid-brain may continue to provide feelings and regulate autonomic physical functions. To be truly Homo sapiens we must be sapient, however minimally. Only this trait or capability is necessary to all of the other traits which go into the fullness of humanness. (1974, 6)

Fletcher described the persistently unconscious patient as dead, although he took pains to point out that death is contingent on a diagnosis of *permanent* unconsciousness[5]:

The "vegetable" patient, no matter how many spontaneous vital functions may be continuing, is dead, a nonperson, but not at the point he appears to be incapable of self-perception or of relational affect—only when neurologic diagnosis determines that cerebral function has ended permanently. (1974, 7)

Grant Gillett has claimed, "A person exists as a continuing subject of consciousness in view of being the subject of a complex of cognitive abilities" (Gillett 1990). A plausible case can be made, he argued, that an individual who has irrevocably lost all capacity for consciousness is dead, and "no longer a person at all" (Gillett 1990, 181).

The nature of cognitive capacities constitutive of consciousness makes an individual a being to whom things matter or 'a locus of ethical value'. These features of a person's existence are dependent

[5] As noted in chapters 1 and 2, the term *persistent vegetative state* is outdated and does not, by definition, indicate permanent unconsciousness. At the time that Fletcher and other early commentators were writing, it was the only term in use.

upon a certain complexity of appreciation of experience and that is why our ethical concern is undermined where extensive neurological damage has irrevocably obliterated her nature as a subject of consciousness. (198)

Gillett's conclusion that ethical concern is "undermined" is interesting, as it implies that it is misguided or a mistake to have ethical concerns about the unconscious individual, much like we might think it's a mistake to worry about the feelings of a toaster or a bicycle or a bacterium.

Jeff McMahan has described the unconscious human as a living *organism*, but a dead *person*:

When those parts of the brain in which consciousness and mental activity are realized are destroyed or rendered irreversibly nonfunctional, the mind ceases to exist—that is, the person dies. . . . In many cases in which a patient enters a persistent vegetative state, what has happened is that the person has died or ceased to exist while the organism, sustained by the operations of the brain stem, remains alive. (1995)

According to these proponents of the General Consciousness Criterion, an individual who loses the capacity for consciousness loses their personhood (or for Fletcher, more crudely, their humanity). For Gillett and McMahan, the loss of mental life or complexity entails the loss of personhood. These notions persisted well after the persistent and permanent VS were differentiated in 1994, and even after the MCS was defined and described in 2002. For example, Ravelingien et al. held that

one could argue that even the term "patient" is inappropriate in relation to the condition, because the word generally refers to a living person, while a body in PVS has permanently lost all forms of personhood. . . . To be a person at minimum requires the capacity for cognitive and affective mental functioning, which is inextricably bound with the notion of awareness. The parts of the brain that are crucial in terms of the mind and to sentient existence are irreversibly lost in a PVS body. (2004, 95)

These claims align with some common folk intuitions about DoCs. In the public imagination, unconscious "vegetative" humans frequently occupy some intermediate space, not-quite-human, not-quite-persons, not-quite-alive. For example, a physician referred to a patient as a "slab of meat" and said "I will not keep a slab of meat, that's all he will be, a slab of meat alive in my room, I won't do that, that's undignified" (quoted in Kitzinger and Kitzinger, 2014). Another doctor referred to a colleague in a vegetative state as "lying in an open grave" and suffering "the ultimate curse" (Crisci 1995). A family member suggested that their relative lacked a mind: "There's a case there and somebody's taken the motherboard out" (quoted in Holland, Kitzinger, and Kitzinger, 2014). Another suggested his mother was no longer alive: "Essentially, she's a cadaver with a heartbeat."[6]

7.2.2 The Particular Consciousness Criterion

Moreover, due to lack of memory, it would be impossible for you to remember that you ever enjoyed yourself, and for any pleasure to survive from one moment to the next, since it would leave no memory. But, not possessing right judgment, you would not realize that you are enjoying yourself even while you do, and, being unable to calculate, you could not figure out any future pleasures for yourself. You would thus not live a human life but the life of a

---

[6] From my case notes for a hospital ethics consultation.

mollusk or one of those creatures in shells that live in the
sea.... But is this a life worth choosing? (Plato 1997)[7]

In *Philebus,* Plato, arguing against Philebus and Protarchus (who
maintain that the best human life is a life of pleasure and enjoy-
ment), sets up a dichotomy between a life of pleasure without
knowledge and a life of knowledge without pleasure. The former,
he argues, would not be a life worthy of a human, but neither would
the latter life be good. The good life, he concludes, would be one
that contains both pleasure and knowledge.

Fletcher went beyond his claim that unconscious individuals,
lacking neocortical function, are dead. He made clear that not just
any neocortical function will do. His view on those with cognitive
and intellectual disabilities, for example, is that "any individual
of the species *Homo sapiens* who falls below the I.Q. 40-mark in
a standard Stanford-Binet test . . . is questionably a person; below
the 20-mark, not a person" (Fletcher 1972, 1). To my knowledge,
he is the only bioethicist to link moral status to one's score on the
notoriously biased Stanford-Binet Intelligence Scale. For Fletcher,
a human with a cognitive impairment is not worthy of being called
a person.

Fletcher didn't consider the value of a rational life without
pleasures, nor was he familiar with the MCS, which was unknown at the time he declared humans with low IQ scores to be
nonpersons. But the MCS might well be the kind of condition in
which there is sentience, and capacities for physical and emotional
feeling (that is, phenomenal consciousness), without sophisticated
cognition or self-awareness. Plato might have thought individuals
in the MCS live shellfish-like lives, disconnected from a persisting

---

[7] Plato was no doubt unaware that some mollusks, especially octopuses with their
large and distributed brains, seem to live rather rich and interesting lives. For more on
octopuses, animal minds, and consciousness, I commend the reader to Peter Godfrey-
Smith's wonderful books, *Other Minds: The Octopus, the Sea, and the Origins of
Consciousness* and *Metazoa: Animal Life and the Birth of the Mind.*

self—lives not worth choosing or living. Fletcher would have said simply that they're not persons.

Neil Levy and Julian Savulescu (Levy and Savulescu 2009; Levy 2009) have offered a more nuanced and detailed account of the relationship between consciousness and moral status. They distinguished between different types of consciousness, using Block's Access/Phenomenal consciousness framework, and claimed that it is *self-consciousness*, which requires access consciousness, that matters for personhood. Phenomenal consciousness refers to the qualitative character or feel, the *what it's likeness,* of conscious experience. Minimally, it requires sentience. Access consciousness, by contrast, describes a state in which information is available for rational control and is accessible to decision-making, planning, and volition. In TFAHs, access and phenomenal consciousness co-occur, along with the "wakeful awareness" that is the clinical diagnostic feature of consciousness. In DoC patients in whom some of these types of consciousness might dissociate, Levy and Savulescu maintained that there are important moral distinctions that depend on the type of consciousness in question.

> Consciousness is closely linked to the moral status of those capable of experiencing it, but the different kinds of consciousness underlie different kinds of moral value. Phenomenal consciousness is sufficient to make its bearer a moral *patient. . . .* To be a moral patient is to be a being whose welfare matters, whose welfare must be taken into account when we decide what to do. To be phenomenally conscious makes one a moral patient because a phenomenally conscious being can experience states that have qualities of aversiveness (like pain or boredom) or of pleasantness (like joy); these states matter intrinsically. (2009, 366)

However, Levy and Savulescu describe moral patiency as a "low grade of moral status," akin to what is accorded to nonhuman animals. On their view, moral patients matter, and we ought not to cause them pain without good reason. But moral patients lack an interest in continuing to live, and thus lack a right to life, so we have no positive reason to maintain them "in being." This would include conscious patients like those in the MCS, who experience transitory and fluctuating awareness that is not sufficient, on this view, to underwrite personhood. For a right to life, one needs to be "capable of very sophisticated mental states that have an ineliminably temporal component" (Levy and Savulescu 2009, 367). Full moral status, they argued, requires that how one's life goes and the satisfaction of one's interests matter to *oneself*, and all this requires "very sophisticated cognitive abilities, such as an ability to conceive of oneself as a being persisting through time, to recall one's past, to plan, and to have preferences for how one's life goes" (Levy and Savulescu 2009, 367). It requires, in other words, Lockean personal identity, and what Levy and Savulescu called "diachronic access consciousness":

> It is the connectedness and continuity of one's mental states that underwrite *personhood*, in one central sense of the word; it is insofar as each of us is a single being across (relatively long) stretches of time that we count as moral persons.
>
> But the abilities that underlie moral personhood and full moral status are abilities that require *access* consciousness, not phenomenal consciousness. Information must be sufficiently available for rational thought and deliberation in order for a being to be able to have future-oriented desires or to conceive of itself as persisting in time. (2009, 367)

Locke's metaphysical claims about persons and personal identity are transmogrified into normative claims about who matters. It's not clear, however, why metaphysical persons with personal identity should matter *morally*, or matter more than someone who lacks the mental capacities needed for diachronic personal identity, all else being equal.[8] For Levy and Savulescu, it matters that one has interests, but not just any interests. A sentient creature capable of experiencing pain, for example, might have interests in avoiding pain because pain is unpleasant and aversive.[9] But only creatures with diachronic access consciousness—a persisting sense of self-identity—can have the kinds of interests in, and preferences about, how their lives go *over time*, and not just *right now*. Those are the interests that make one a person with a right to life, on their view.

Joshua Shepherd, by contrast, has argued that *phenomenal* consciousness—the capacity for phenomenal states, is the relevant feature of entities with moral status. Phenomenal states, he argued, are the condition for being a bearer of non-derivative value:

> An entity E bears moral status if and only if E bears non-derivative value. Moreover, the particular reasons we have to treat E in various ways are largely a function of [the] way E bears whatever non-derivative value she does. (2018, 16)[10]

On Shepherd's view, entities have moral status by virtue of their essential properties, and the relevant properties are the ones by virtue of which the entity *bears* non-derivative value. That is, things are intrinsically valuable *to* the entity because the entity has phenomenal consciousness. There is something it is like for the entity to have experiences. Experiences are happy and sad, pleasant and painful, positive and negative. They have non-derivative value because they

---

[8] It bears saying that the necessity of consciousness and sophisticated cognition for personhood, as described by Fletcher, Gillett, and Levy and Savulescu, excludes many humans, including infants, and some with cognitive or intellectual disabilities, advanced dementia, and those with DoCs. Levy and Savulescu noted that some apes would likely count as persons according to their view.

[9] It's not clear that all sentient creatures experience pain, or the aversiveness of pain. Sharks do not appear to, and insects don't exhibit the behaviors that typically indicate that one is bothered by an injury that might be painful.

[10] By *non-derivative value* Shepherd meant the value something has on its own or in its own right, rather than the "derivative" value it might have as a thing that accomplishes something else of value. A fragrant, fresh-baked loaf of bread has nonderivative value, but an oven has derivative value as a thing that bakes bread.

have "essentially affective evaluative phenomenal properties," and those properties are present to an entity by virtue of its being phenomenally conscious. The value of experiences may depend in part on the cognitive sophistication of the bearer, but that is not to say that simpler creatures value *less* than more cognitively sophisticated creatures. The important point is that to be a bearer of nonderivative value at all requires phenomenal consciousness, and thus moral status depends on phenomenal consciousness.

Both conclusions here hinge on having interests and assume that one can value or disvalue certain states of affairs. As I have argued, even unconscious individuals can have interests, although not in the same way that you or I have interests. Our interests can be experienced as desires or preferences we have now (or remembered as past preferences). Our interests are in an important sense flexible and mutable and can respond to what happens in our lives. Some of the things that happen in our lives might make us value continued life less (experiencing intractable pain or refractory depression), while some might make us value it more. The question is whether merely having access consciousness in the absence of phenomenal consciousness would be enough for having interests (and moral status). Levy and Savulescu claimed that moral patients—those with phenomenal consciousness but not diachronic access consciousness—have a low-grade moral status but lack an interest in continued life. I find myself agreeing with Plato (which is a strange sensation) that a continuing, self-aware life without phenomenal consciousness would not be a good life and might well be one I'd have no interest in continuing. But that's not our question. Our question is whether the entity lacking either phenomenal or diachronic access consciousness is a person.

For Levy and Savulescu, only entities with access consciousness can have an interest in continued life. Can an entity with *only* access consciousness have the capacity to value their life and continued life? That is, might one value life without that life containing valued experiences? As Levy and Savulescu noted, phenomenal states of pleasure and pain have *intrinsic* value. Would a life without any phenomenal states have intrinsic value? Shepherd would deny that it does. A Utilitarian ought to deny that it does. Perhaps Levy and Savulescu, although they conceived of moral patients with phenomenal but not access consciousness (e.g., MCS patients), didn't imagine a realistic scenario in which an entity has access, but not phenomenal, consciousness.[11] Moreover, because it is self-consciousness that makes one a person, they might well think that absent self-consciousness, phenomenal consciousness would be in some important sense different or diminished. Without a sense of self-identity, a pain or a pleasure might be present in my conscious experience without it identifiably being *my* pain or *my* pleasure. Shepherd denied that self-consciousness is "especially closely related to evaluative experiential capacities" (Shepherd 2018, 98). But certainly it's true that someone else's pains and pleasures affect me quite differently than my own do. If my phenomenal experiences are in some sense dissociated from *me*, then perhaps the me of which I am not self-aware would be capable of bearing less value. On the other hand, lacking the ability to think about, or to make sense of, a pain, or to recognize its temporality—say the pain of childbirth, or of a pan-galactic gargleblaster—might well make that pain more

---

[11] Such entities are known in philosophy of mind as p-zombies, or philosophical zombies. They are essentially phenomenally empty inside. They can sense and think, but there is nothing it is like for them to taste a ripe peach or hear music. There is no what-it's-likeness of those experiences, although from the outside, p-zombies look and behave just like conscious creatures. There is a question whether p-zombies are possible—could a p-zombie look and behave just like a conscious animal? There are documented cases of individuals who lack some phenomenal experiences. A Scottish woman named Jo Cameron has pain asymbolia caused by a rare genetic mutation (Habib et al. 2019). Cameron, now in her seventies, has never experienced pain as painful, and describes giving birth as feeling "like a tickle" (Murphy 2019). She frequently accidentally burns herself as well (pain, although unpleasant, is useful—it helps us avoid things that will cause damage to our bodies), and so she doesn't behave like someone who feels pain. For most of us, the pain of a burn is very unpleasant. It has a particular qualitative feeling, unlike, say, the pleasant taste of chocolate or the prickly sensation of goosebumps. Cameron's unusual behavior suggests that a p-zombie wouldn't behave just like a phenomenally conscious human.

immediately experienced.[12] In that case, phenomenal consciousness without access consciousness might well result in more value (or disvalue), rather than less.

The Particular Consciousness Criterion is more fine-grained than the General Consciousness Criterion. It handles some of the edge cases, like the MCS, with more subtlety than the General Consciousness Criterion does. It does not, I think, make a better case for thinking that a Consciousness Criterion for moral status or personhood works.

7.3 Consciousness Criterion or Capacities Criterion?

One question that wants answering at this point is whether consciousness (or a particular type of consciousness) matters intrinsically or matters instrumentally. If the latter, then there are further questions: What capacities or functions undergirded by consciousness matter for moral status? And why not cut to the chase and focus on those capacities instead?

Let's cut to the chase. I'll call an instrumental consciousness criterion a Capacities Criterion. A Capacities Criterion is frequently a list (sometimes quite extensive and detailed) of the capacities of beings with moral status.

Tom Regan called his criterion for moral status the "subject-of-a-life criterion." Being a subject-of-a-life, he argued, "involves more than being alive and more than merely being conscious" (Regan 2004, 243).

---

[12] Specker-Sullivan's discussion of "pure experience" is again relevant here. Pure experience is an experience that is:

> immediate, without any cognition, deliberation, or judgment. . . . The absence of ownership of the experience and cognition concerning the content of the experience signifies that this is a level of consciousness that precedes the differentiation of subject and object; it is an objectless experience, but it is also a subjectless experience. (Specker Sullivan 2018, 111)

Individuals are subjects-of-a-life if they have beliefs and desires; perceptions, memory, and a sense of the future, including their own future; an emotional life together with feelings of pleasure and pain; preference- and welfare-interests; the ability to initiate action in pursuit of their desires and goals; a psychophysical identity over time; and an individual welfare in the sense that their experiential life fares well or ill for them, logically independently of their utility for others and logically independently of their being the object of anyone else's interest. Those who satisfy the subject-of-a-life criterion themselves have a distinctive kind of value— inherent value—and are not to be viewed or treated as mere receptacles. (2004, 243)

Regan claimed that his subject-of-a-life criterion is not explicitly a consciousness criterion—it requires *more* than consciousness. The requirements are quite demanding and include having a sense of the future and of oneself as a self persisting in the future. If Levy and Savulescu are right, that requires self-consciousness and diachronic access consciousness. But Regan's subjects-of-a-life also need phenomenal consciousness for feelings of pleasure and pain and for emotions.

For Regan, both moral agents and moral patients are subjects-of-a-life and have equal inherent (or categorical) value. That is, moral status does not admit of degrees. We have direct duties to both moral agents and moral patients. Not all living things are subjects-of-a-life, but it is also the case that some entities that are not subjects-of-a-life might still have inherent value, for the subject-of-a-life criterion is a *sufficient* criterion, not a *necessary* one. As a sufficient condition, it

does not preclude the possibility that those humans and animals who fail to meet the subject-of-a-life criterion nonetheless have inherent value. . . . It remains possible that animals that are conscious but not capable of acting intentionally, or, say, permanently comatose human beings, might nonetheless be viewed as having inherent value. . . . However, it must be said that it is radically unclear how the attribution of inherent value to these individuals can be made intelligible and nonarbitrary. (2004, 246)[13]

Regan's admission of unconscious humans and animals who lack some of the capacities he includes in his criterion is somewhat grudging. It seems clear that entities without brains—those underappreciated shellfish again—or without typically functioning brains that support consciousness cannot satisfy his demanding criterion, and so their inherent value must be grounded in something else. For that reason, although he claims that his criterion is sufficient but not necessary, and he specifies the exact capacities and abilities that satisfy his criterion, it still looks and quacks like a Consciousness Criterion. Call it a Consciousness + Capacities Criterion.

Warren, in specifying the five capacities or "traits which are most central to the concept of personhood or humanity in the moral sense" (Warren 1973), put consciousness at the top of the list, and it is apparent consciousness is necessary (but not sufficient) for the other four traits.[14] A conscious creature (an infant, or someone in the MCS) might still be unable to perform most of the other functions Warren lists, such as reasoning or communicating. Warren added that, minimally, consciousness and reasoning (which she defines as the *developed* capacity to solve new and relatively complex problems) alone may be *sufficient* for personhood,

---

[13] Regan was troubled by the implication that some nonconscious, non-subjects-of-a-life natural objects, like trees and lakes, might have inherent value.

[14] Warren's five traits are: consciousness (of objects and events external and/or internal to the being), and in particular the capacity to feel pain; reasoning (the *developed* capacity to solve new and relatively complex problems); self-motivated activity (activity that is relatively independent of either genetic or direct external control); the capacity to communicate, by whatever means, messages of an indefinite variety of types, that is, not just with an indefinite number of possible contents, but on indefinitely many possible topics; and the presence of self-concepts, and self-awareness, either individual or racial, or both (Warren 1973).

but any creature possessing none of the capacities or traits cannot be a person. "Full-blooded personhood," for Warren, requires the capacity for moral agency (Warren 1997), that is, the capacity to reason according to, and be motivated by, morality. Here Warren diverged from Regan, for whom moral agents and moral patients have equal moral worth. Warren's criteria taken together can also be designated as a Consciousness + Capacities Criterion.

Warren identified the relevant traits or capacities that typical persons have that are not shared by contested persons. This approach is a common one for those who go to the trouble of developing and defending a Capacities Criterion for moral status or personhood, whether the contested entities are fetuses, humans with DoCs (or other "marginal cases"), or nonhumans (animals, robots, AIs, extraterrestrials, etc.). It's an approach that Shepherd described as working backward from paradigmatic persons to establish the grounds of moral status so that it can then be determined whether any other entities qualify for moral status (Shepherd 2018). It looks for X by looking at the capacities that uncontested persons have. The problem with this approach occurs right at the ground—establishing what capacities undergird moral status or personhood in TFAHs. TFAHs have many different capacities, traits, and characteristics, some of which appear quite trivial with respect to mattering morally. Needless to say, in human history many of those traits have been employed to deny full personhood or moral status to some humans, and to underwrite genocide, slavery, and other atrocities. (Some of those traits include skin color, sex, geographic and ethnic origins, developmental age, sexual orientation, and physical and cognitive capacities.) We should tread carefully in establishing criteria for personhood lest we arbitrarily declare relevant just those capacities or traits found in TFAHs (where what is considered typical is restricted to a narrow range) but not found in non-typically functioning humans.

In principle, there seems to be no reason to adopt a Consciousness Criterion if what we're really interested in are other mental or cognitive capacities like the ability to feel, think, remember, communicate, or to connect one's past, present, and future into a unitary self. It's not obvious that all of those capacities require awareness—some frequently operate below the level of conscious awareness. (Although that does not prove that consciousness "under the hood," as it were, is not still present in the kinds of creatures who have those capacities.) As is demonstrated by some patients who recover consciousness, their other capacities might or might not be affected. Some, like Terry Wallis, lose the ability to experience the passage of time, and remain fixed in the past, as it were. Some have amnesia or aphasia. Having regained consciousness, they satisfy the General Consciousness Criterion. We don't generally debate whether an amnesiac has a right to life, even if they've lost the connecting threads of their life.[15] That suggests it's still just the fact of consciousness rather than capacities that require consciousness that seems to matter. But capacities criteria, if they describe only the *sufficient* conditions for moral status, can, as Warren and Regan did, allow that some capacities can be absent in an entity with moral status. Absent consciousness, however, having sufficient capacities

---

[15] K.C. is an amnesiac with a remarkable history and condition. He suffered three head injuries during his life. The first, when he was 16, happened when a hay bale fell on his head. The second occurred when his homemade dune buggy collided with another vehicle. The third, a motorcycle crash, left him comatose for 3 days and permanently amnesic. Any details of personal experiences (episodic memory) were lost to his mind, and he had no ability to commit new information to memory. According to the researchers who studied him for decades, "K.C. lacks 'autonoetic' consciousness, which refers to the subjective awareness of not only remembering the past but also thinking about the future" (Rosenbaum et al. 2005, 993):

> The events surrounding a recent fall at his family's cottage that resulted in several operations to repair a shattered knee, a cast from waist to toe, and his residing in the main floor living room with crutches for over 6 months, are similarly as good as gone. Each time he is told of September 11, he expresses the same horror and disbelief as someone hearing of the news for the very first time. (Rosenbaum et al. 2005, 994)

K.C. is not entirely lacking in access consciousness. He is capable of performing activities of daily living, retains skills he learned before his motorcycle accident, and at the time of the report in 2005, had a job sorting books in a library. Yet he lacks diachronic access consciousness, the self that connects all the experiences of his life. It seems quite implausible to suggest that he is not a person.

of the kind Warren and Regan described would be out of reach, so at bottom, their Capacities + Consciousness Criterion apparently reduces to a Consciousness Criterion.

A capacities-only criterion that named *necessary* capacities would have different implications than a Consciousness Criterion. One could claim that individuals who have lost, say, the capacity for autobiographical memory or autonomy are no longer persons, even if they are still conscious. Brain injuries and disorders can result in the loss of various capacities without the loss of consciousness. One could certainly be conscious and lack some or all of the potential personal capacities listed above—newborn infants and some individuals with severe cognitive disabilities might lack some or all of them. If it is difficult to reduce personhood to the capacity for consciousness, it will be even more difficult to reduce it to other capacities seemingly instantiated in/supported by selective regions of the brain, or, put less reductively, undergirded by other cognitive capacities, not least of which because individuals without select capacities could still function in ways plausibly similar to TFAHs.

If we dig in our heels and insist that a Consciousness Criterion is right, we can argue that none of the morally relevant capacities can be realized without consciousness. Self- and access consciousness are required for autonomy, memory, rationality, self-awareness and the like, and those capacities are person-making. Consciousness, then, is a necessary property for the possession of other properties or capacities necessary for moral status. That gets us to "consciousness is necessary for personhood," but with a few steps in between. We might think, then, that while consciousness is not itself a *moral* property of persons, it is a necessary precondition—the substrate—for having certain morally relevant capacities that amount to personhood. Problematically, these properties require more than mere consciousness, as evidenced, for example, by the fact that there are conscious individuals (like K.C., discussed in note 15) who lack autobiographical memory due to brain injuries, or amnestic mild cognitive impairment, or Alzheimer's dementia, or who lack autonomy due to frontotemporal dementia.

When the marginal cases under consideration involve DoCs, the salient feature seems to be the *loss* of consciousness. That's an ad hoc reason, but not a compelling reason for thinking consciousness matters. We could just as easily shift our attention to disorders of other types, such as amnesia or dementia, or, as seen in the abortion and animal ethics literatures, cognitive sophistication and psychological complexity. It might feel less right to say that the granny who has lost her autobiographical memory to dementia, but who still laughs and sings and enjoys chocolate cake, is no longer a person, and more right to say that the unconscious 28-year-old who can't do any of those things is no longer a person. That it seems so certainly says something about our intuitions about personhood and consciousness, but our intuitions are at best inconsistent.

Being a person (or having moral status) is a *moral* property of entities. Consciousness is not a moral property. The kinds of mental capacities that are necessary for personhood on the Particular Consciousness Criterion view—such as autobiographical memory, diachronic identity, the ability to engage in rational deliberation about one's actions, and to have experiences with subjective qualities—require consciousness, but not consciousness alone (or access or phenomenal consciousness alone). Personhood, then, is not reducible to consciousness or to particular capacities undergirded by consciousness.

7.4 Moral Agents and Moral Patients

Consider two candidates for *moral properties*. Moral agency is a moral property of some entities, those capable of being sufficiently guided and motivated by, and of responding to and acting on, moral reasons (that is, some conception of what is good or right). As Regan defined them,

> Moral agents are individuals who have a variety of sophisti-
> cated abilities, including in particular the ability to bring impar-
> tial moral principles to bear on the determination of what, all
> considered, morally ought to be done and, having made this de-
> termination, to freely choose or fail to choose to act as morality,
> as they conceive it, requires. (2004, 151)

So. That's a lot. Lots of humans won't cut the mustard, moral agent-
wise. Moral patients are entities who are the subjects of some (as
yet unspecified) moral obligations or duties on the part of moral
agents.[16] They "lack the prerequisites that would enable them to
control their own behavior in ways that would make them morally
accountable for what they do" (Regan 2004, 152). If possession of
moral properties is necessary for moral status, then moral patiency
and moral agency are candidate properties for having moral status.

Moral agency is a moral property of TFAHs. It requires any
number of other properties or capacities: autonomy, rationality,
and self-awareness among them. It's hard to conceive of an unconscious creature exercising any of these capacities or being a moral
agent (or any other kind of agent). But, of course, there are conscious creatures—conscious humans—who are also not moral
agents. The defining feature of moral agency as a capacity is that
it gives us the ability to take on the responsibilities and duties that
moral agents have. As Uncle Ben might say, "With moral agency
comes great responsibility." For this reason, we don't hold infants
morally responsible—they simply lack the capacities needed to
be moral agents. They neither can be moved by moral reasons nor

---

[16] We face the same criterion problem with moral patients if their status must be reducible to nonmoral properties or capacities. Sentience is frequently cited as the criterion for moral patiency. I'll leave unresolved the question of what criteria pick out
moral patients beyond identifying them as *nonmoral agents to whom moral agents have
obligations*. I'm sympathetic to Hale's "deontological" discussion of moral considerability
in which it is conceived as an obligation of moral agents. That is, it is not incumbent
on other entities to show why they deserve moral consideration or to offer up reasons
for considering them within a moral frame. Rather, it is one of the obligations of moral
agents that they morally consider other entities. (Hale 2011).

can they act on them. But if all we mean by "moral status" is moral agency, we can bypass consciousness and just say that only moral agents are persons. So, we could argue that:

All and only moral agents are persons
P is a moral agent
Therefore, P is a person

We can't make the move from *P is a moral agent* to *P is a person* without the first premise, that is, without assuming that moral agents are persons. We might have reasons to think that *all* moral agents are persons, but less solid reasons to think that *only* moral agents are persons. If there are nonmoral agents who matter morally to any degree, then moral status and moral agency are not coextensive or synonymous.[17] Moral patients are nonmoral agents who matter morally, so moral agency and moral status are not coextensive or synonymous. The difference between moral agents and moral patients is that, while both have moral status, only the former also have moral obligations to other agents and patients. Moral patients do not have such obligations because they are not capable of having them. As Godfrey Tangwa has said, moral agents "are not morally special, they are morally liable" (Tangwa 2000, 40). And as Alastair Norcross has argued, being a moral agent is simply a different property from having moral status (Norcross 2004). That is, moral agents don't matter *more* than moral patients. Warren, by contrast, claimed that only with moral agency comes "full-blooded personhood."

Moral agency requires a relatively sophisticated kind of rationality. Locke recognized that moral agency requires diachronic

---

[17] Likewise, if there are moral agents who do not matter morally, then they are not synonymous. The moral status or personhood of nonhuman animals is contested despite growing evidence of the moral agency (e.g., altruism, sensitivity to justice and fairness) of some species, including dogs and nonhuman primates, and the possibility that moral agency may admit of degrees (see note 2, this chapter).

consciousness, the ability to mentally plan and connect through time one's actions and the later effects of those actions. Levy and Savulescu argued that to have a right to life, one must also have an interest in continued life, which also requires rather sophisticated cognitive abilities and self-consciousness. I'm not convinced that having rights requires any sort of mental sophistication at all. Young infants don't have self-consciousness or cognitive sophistication or a sense of themselves as persisting selves, and some persons may never develop those capacities, or may lose them. Yet they may still have moral rights without having corresponding interests they can conceive of. (Infants don't understand lungs either, but they still have interests in the good functioning of their lungs, and rights against having their lungs taken from them.) The right to life is not different. The moral property that clearly requires some mental sophistication is moral agency. In humans, and within Western philosophical traditions, moral agency involves being able to understand, recognize, and respect the rights of others, and to act as morality requires. If only moral agents can have rights, then the world is full of creatures, including many humans, who do not and cannot have rights, and who do not matter morally. That would be a radical revision of the way moral rights and rights-bearers are understood, and it would exclude many more than those who are unconscious and minimally conscious. It would also conflate moral agency and personhood, and it would mistake moral agency for an entitlement of the cognitively sophisticated rather than a responsibility.

But wait, you might be saying. Children and infants are not moral agents, but they have the *potential* to be moral agents in the future, and so they have rights. Someone who is permanently unconscious has no such potential, and likewise someone with advanced dementia. The abortion ethics literature is replete with discussions about potentiality as a criterion of personhood, and I won't rehearse those arguments here. The difficulty of advancing this claim for our present purposes is not so much that individuals with DoCs lack the potential for moral agency, but rather that *all of us* have the potential to lose moral agency and to become, at that point, nonpersons. Potentiality, if it matters, should cut both ways. If the mere potential to *become a person* matters morally, so should the mere potential to *become a nonperson*. The discussion at hand concerns whether DoC patients, who have lost the capacity to be moral agents are *no longer* persons. If merely having the potential to lose moral agency matters for personhood and having rights, then none of us are persons, and none of us have rights.

There's another wrinkle. If moral patients are not rights-bearers, then the moral obligations of moral agents to them require explanation. One could deny that moral agents have duties to moral patients. Warren denied this when, faced with the implication that her criteria for personhood would permit infanticide, she argued that others (persons, parents, society) would be displeased if infants they cared about were killed. Immanuel Kant, similarly, argued that shooting a dog would not harm the dog, but would harm other members of the moral community who had some interest in the dog. These *might* be plausible accounts of the wrong of destroying a tree or a work of art, but they are not adequate accounts of the harm or wrong of killing infants and dogs. (Levy and Savulescu didn't claim that moral patients have no rights. They claimed they have limited rights.)

But, assume for the sake of argument that it's true that psychologically simple creatures like human infants or dogs lack diachronic access consciousness, lack a sense of a persistent self, and don't care how their lives go, or whether they continue to live. (The reader might want to lodge a protest here and deny that any of this applies to dogs. I agree, but bear with me.) I think it is likely true that very young infants (and probably very young puppies) have none of these mental properties. What is the moral relevance of these properties, and what do they tell us about the moral property of having/not having moral status with respect to infants or puppies? That is, why is the *description* of infants and puppies *prescriptive*? It isn't, for all the reasons discussed above.

7.4.1 Interests, Harms, and Rights

Instead of claiming that moral status is reducible to nonmoral properties, we could follow James Rachels in saying that certain properties or capacities of creatures make them vulnerable to certain corresponding kinds of harm. That bypasses moral status and explains rights in terms of morally relevant properties. Taking an interest-based view of rights thus connects rights to preferences (or interests). On this view, rights are not free-floating, but correspond to the interests of the rights-bearer. A right to liberty, for example, requires that the bearer be autonomous and have an interest in liberty.

> There is no characteristic, or reasonably small set of characteristics, that sets some creatures apart from others as meriting respectful treatment. That is the wrong way to think about the relation between an individual's characteristics and how he or she may be treated. Instead we have an array of characteristics and an array of treatments, with each characteristic relevant to justifying some types of treatment but not others.
>
> If asked, toward whom is it appropriate to direct fundamental moral consideration? we could reply: It is appropriate to direct fundamental moral consideration toward any individual who has any of the indefinitely long list of characteristics that constitute morally good reasons why he or she should or should not be treated in any of the various ways in which individuals may be treated. (2004, 169–170)

One benefit of this way of thinking about moral consideration is that it doesn't grant enhanced standing to some by virtue of their characteristics or traits, or by virtue of being moral agents. Those theories run aground on devising non-arbitrary justifications for that enhanced standing. As Rachels argued, "Autonomy and self-consciousness are not ethical superqualities that entitle the bearer to every possible kind of favorable treatment. . . . They are relevant to some types of treatment but not to others" (Rachels 2004, 167). Rachels' view also has the benefit of bypassing the problem with theories that posit criteria for moral status, which is that they must justify those moral criteria in terms of nonmoral characteristics or traits of entities. Rachels, on the other hand, linked types of treatment directly to nonmoral but morally relevant characteristics—for example, sentient creatures are susceptible to pain, and that gives us a moral reason to not cause them pain.

Moreover, this approach resolves the puzzle about why moral agents *should* have moral duties to nonmoral agents, and not merely duties to other moral agents not to cause harm to the things (babies, puppies) they happen to care about. Moral agents have duties to moral patients because the latter have, for example, rights corresponding to their vulnerabilities to physical and psychological injury, and they can be wronged and morally injured. When a dog is neglected and starved, we think both that the dog has been physically harmed and that there is a moral wrong done to the dog. The dog has been caused to suffer and has been denied that to which dogs have a right—sustenance—for no good reason. That moral injury can only be inflicted by a moral agent, one who has moral responsibilities and duties of care to others. Having duties and responsibilities is what sets moral agents apart from moral patients, because moral agents are the kinds of creatures who can be saddled with duties and responsibilities. As Norcross argued, "What grounds moral agency is simply different from what grounds moral standing as a patient" (Norcross 2004, 243), so there is no puzzle about how moral agents *and* moral patients can have rights, or how moral agents can have duties to moral patients.

One possible outcome of the view that one's rights correspond to one's interests is that creatures who lack an interest in continued life cannot have a right to life (as Levy and Savulescu claim). Much depends, in that case, on what is required to "have an interest" in something. Very many interests do not require having sophisticated understanding of concepts. Orcas at SeaWorld and elephants in zoos and the dog living at the end of a chain have an interest in liberty even if they have no concept of "liberty." A dog can have an interest in living even without having a sophisticated understanding of philosophical concepts like the persistence of personal identity, because a dog can have goals and projects that extend into the future even if "future" is not a concept they have (*I'm going to keep digging that hole. I'm going to go see if it's dinnertime*). So, I'm skeptical that having an interest in continuing to live requires having a sophisticated conception of one's self, being able to formulate a thought like "I'd rather like it if I continued to live," or even having a psychologically continuous sense of self. I'm skeptical that an MCS patient or a VS/UWS patient doesn't have interests in life continuing or not. As I argued in Chapter 6, unconscious persons do have interests in what happens to them and how their lives go, and in that case, can have the same interests and right to life that a conscious person has.[18]

Psychologically simple creatures like infants and puppies can be harmed in some ways (e.g., by being starved) while psychologically complex creatures like TFAHs can be harmed in other ways. That's merely a description of how one's level of psychological complexity

---

[18] I'm not committed to the existence of a "right to life" per se. It's too crude a concept, as it is often used or understood. An individual's desire to live or interest in living is morally relevant, and so, too, is their interest in not continuing to live, but as I have argued, one need not be conscious or aware in the moment to have those interests. I address the so-called right to life because it is frequently invoked in discussions about continuing life-sustaining treatment for DoC patients.

makes one vulnerable or susceptible to different kinds of harms. If we think there is a moral duty to avoid harming others (which is a pretty standard moral view I won't bother defending), then our specific duties will vary depending on the creature we are dealing with. But that implies nothing about the value or status of that creature. Psychologically simple and complex creatures are equally susceptible to certain kinds of harm. We can harm and wrong them both by, for example, starving them.[19] We can also harm and wrong a psychologically complex being by, for example, making it impossible for them to fulfill a lifelong goal, or by hurting someone else they care about, or by destroying a family heirloom they cherish. Being susceptible to *more* kinds of harm is an odd candidate for *enhanced* moral status. Having access consciousness, being psychologically complex, and self-conscious, then, are odd candidates for *enhanced* moral status.

The question of whether someone has an interest in some state of affairs *S*, as a way of determining if they matter morally, gets it backward. Having an interest in *S* tells us whether moral *agents* have moral duties with respect to *S* (to bring about *S*, to not bring about *S*, etc.). By the time we get to that level of consideration, we should already know that the subject of *S* matters morally. If they don't, then *S* can be of little concern. Thus, whether a VS/UWS patient has an interest in continued life should matter to moral agents only if the VS/UWS patient matters morally.

---

[19] Perhaps starving is an invidious example. Artificial nutrition and hydration (ANH) is one form of life-sustaining treatment (LST) that can be withheld from individuals with DoCs (who are frequently not dependent on a ventilator). It is commonly denied that it is a harm to withdraw ANH from an unconscious individual because they do not feel pain or distress. The harm of withdrawing LST then, would be that they eventually die, and it is denied that dying is a harm to someone whose life is not a benefit. One can agree with all of this without also agreeing that unconscious individuals are not persons. Indeed, if it's relevant whether or not someone can be harmed by some action, we have already admitted that it matters morally what we do, and that they matter morally.

7.4.2 The Burdens of Moral Agents

Benjamin Hale has argued that the way to think about moral considerability is not in terms of the qualities or capacities of moral patients, but in terms of the obligations that rational moral agents have to them.

> I propose that, rather than focusing exclusively on the attributes or capacities of other beings as qualifiers for moral patienthood, the question is more comprehensible as uniquely limited to whether and why an agent has responsibility to assess a narrower or wider set of considerations regarding entities in the world. (2011, 38)

One benefit of this approach is that we have a pretty good idea of what moral agency requires. A typical Western view is that it requires rationality, autonomy, self-governance, the capacity to consider moral reasons and moral principles, and the capacity to be motivated to act according to those concepts and principles. (There is a good amount of agreement about the needed capacities across other philosophical and cultural traditions that have the concept of moral agency, including those that are less individualistic and less focused on autonomy, such as Confucianism.) These are pretty sophisticated capacities, but as Tangwa noted, moral agents are not morally *special* because they possess these capacities, they are just morally *liable* for what they do, and for what they owe to others.

> What the attributes of self-consciousness, rationality, and freedom of choice do . . . is load the heavy burden of moral liability, culpability, and responsibility on the shoulders of their possessor. (2000, 40)

Norcross described it this way: "Full status as a moral patient is not some kind of reward for moral agency. . . . Humans are subject to moral obligations because they are the kind of creatures who *can* be" (Norcross 2004, 243). Norcross was discussing human obligations to animals as moral patients, but we could just as easily substitute moral agents for humans and say that "*moral agents* are subject to moral obligations because they are the kind of creatures who can be." This is a fruitful approach to thinking about moral status, and one that recognizes that lacking the capacities that enable moral agency does not disqualify an entity from moral considerability, moral status, or personhood. Lacking the capacities for moral agency simply discharges one from the responsibilities of moral agency. In other words, possessing sophisticated rationality and capacities for moral reasoning and self-control, and being self-conscious of oneself as a persisting self, *are* morally relevant. But they are not morally relevant in the way that the General or Particular Consciousness Criterion implies—they pick out moral agents rather than persons, but they do not exclude moral patients from personhood.

7.5 The Epistemic Challenge

Let's suppose that we are willing to ignore all that and commit to the Consciousness Criterion, and maintain that the moral property of mattering morally, or being a person, follows from the nonmoral property of consciousness. We might still challenge the Consciousness Criterion on epistemic grounds.

The question is whether there is a discernible fact of the matter when it comes to consciousness, something on which a moral fact about moral status can be hung. I think there is not. There are two reasons. One is that consciousness is not an identifiable thing, process, capacity, or function. Neural correlates of consciousness, among the holy grails of consciousness studies, are (presumably) things your brain is doing when you are conscious and having conscious states, and not doing when you are not conscious. They are *correlates* of consciousness, not consciousness itself. There is still an inference about consciousness being made. The second reason is related to the first: our ability to determine (or diagnose) who is and who is not conscious is pretty terrible except in standard cases where we can infer it with reasonable certainty based on behaviors like first-person reports.

If there are properties that determine personhood, they ought to withstand a fair amount of scrutiny and be quite certain, given the moral importance of being right about personhood. Suppose we were to say that "all humans are persons." We can be quite certain about who is and who is not human. We have tests. There might be some outliers, such as humanoids that look very much like humans, but are not. Our genetic tests can eliminate them. (Of course, many humanoids are also possibly persons, and humanity, despite its high level of epistemic certainty, is not a *necessary* criterion for personhood.)

Consciousness is not up to the task of determining who can and cannot be a person in the way something like *being human* could be. There are very many conscious creatures in the world, creatures about whom we can verify their consciousness with the same precision that we can verify the consciousness of a TFAH. But TFAHs are the easy cases. Our current ability to identify (or diagnose) consciousness is not very good in the hard cases, and certainly not with a high enough degree of certainty for something as important as having moral status or being a person. The inductive risk is that if we are wrong about who is not a person, there are ethically serious consequences—we may treat someone as if they are not sentient, or are dead, or not a person who matters morally.

McMahan was unmoved by the possibility of being wrong about consciousness. He thought it is "possible in most cases to determine with virtual certainty when recovery is impossible," and he considered the permanently unconscious individual to be dead (McMahan 1998). He allowed for the possibility that "some dim, flickering, rudimentary mode of consciousness might survive cortical death" but thought it a remote possibility. Moreover, he argued,

> It is hard to believe that whatever shadowy, semi-conscious mental activity we might imagine occurring after cortical death could contribute to the good of a person's life. Indeed, there are good reasons for thinking that, for most of us, continued existence as what one commentator called a 'manicured vegetable' would be against our objective interests . . . a possibility of life that could scarcely be worth living. (1998, 259)[20]

McMahan was wrong, of course, about the certainty of diagnosis and prognosis. The high rate of misdiagnosis has been known, and has been virtually unchanged, for four decades. Whether life in something like the MCS is worth living is an entirely different question, but again, here's the rub: if the entity in question does not matter morally, if they are effectively "dead," or a "manicured vegetable," then we need not concern ourselves with whether their life is worth living. It simply would not matter. That we do concern ourselves with whether their life is worth living implies that they do matter morally (unless we are simply making a mistake, as Gillett suggested).

7.5.1 Reducing the Risks

Given our current understanding of consciousness, if we claim that consciousness is *necessary* for moral status, we set the bar too high, epistemically speaking. We are likely to fail to catch (perhaps many) humans who matter morally. Given the inductive risks of being

---

[20] McMahan attributed the "manicured vegetable" line to Ronald Dworkin in *Life's Dominion*. Dworkin actually wrote "scrupulously tended vegetable," one of several instances in the book where he referred to PVS patients as vegetables (Dworkin 1994, 180).

wrong, we should look for a less risky candidate for X. Whatever that criterion is, it ought to satisfy some conditions that reduce the epistemic and ethical risks, and satisfy the Second Principle of Induction. I propose these conditions:

Enduring—A person now would continue to be a person later. Whatever makes them a person will persist. Indeed, when we speak of dead persons, we still think there are some duties owed to them, grounded in respect for persons. When we classify a person as "dead," our duties to them might change, but this is not unusual. Our duties to typical living persons also change with circumstances. The paternalistic protection and care we owe to infants do not persist through adulthood, where they would conflict with respecting autonomy. But our duties to a person with dementia might well include those paternalistic duties of care and protection. Again, the specifics of our duties might change, but if they are grounded in rights and respect for persons, then personhood must persist.

Nonfluctuating—Persons ought not pop in and out of existence every time they fall asleep, or undergo anesthesia, or fall into a coma for some period of time. (Personhood isn't by necessity temporally bounded, so the temporal intervals of consciousness and unconsciousness are irrelevant.) The awareness of those in the MCS is known to fluctuate, but "fluctuate" in practice means only that the *behaviors* from which awareness is inferred fluctuate, and not in the predictable ways of TFAHs. Behaving in nonstandard, atypical ways is a poor correlate of personhood.

Epistemically robust—Given the serious risks of being wrong, we ought to be able to know, with a level of certainty commensurate with the risks, who is and is not a person. This favors having easily verifiable, noncontingent, *sufficient* criteria like "being human" or "being a member of a community with other persons," rather than "having a typically enough functioning brain" or "being conscious."

Consider some necessary conditions of being *human*: conceived of human gametes, born of human parents, having a human genome. This would rule out a humanoid robot like Murderbot, who is constructed of synthetic and organic cloned parts. All of these conditions would be enduring—anyone qualifying as human by satisfying these criteria would not find their status changing. Likewise, they would be nonfluctuating. A human would not cease to be human because they acquire a hip implant, or fall asleep, or inhale a virus. Being human is verifiable and epistemically robust— we could, if we had doubts about those infected with viruses, verify that they are human by checking on the enduring properties. (Still born of human parents—check. Still has a human genome—check.) If having bits of foreign genetic material or metal in one's body is enough to disrupt one's humanity, then not only are there many no-longer-humans among us, but their status is quite contingent—the bits of viral RNA will eventually be gone, and the metal hip could also be removed, thus restoring them to full human status. Until the next virus or bit of pollen invades. If contingent and fluctuating criteria are *necessary* for humanity, then it is difficult to see why being human is meaningful or special. But while being human is verifiable, as a criterion for personhood it may be *sufficient*, but not necessary. Our epistemic standards for what count as *sufficient* criteria can be less demanding than our standards for *necessary* criteria, given the corresponding ethical risks. I suspect there are very many sufficient criteria for personhood, but possibly none that are necessary.

Consciousness is epistemically flimsy, and not a good candidate for a *necessary* criterion of personhood. The problem of misdiagnosis in DoCs has persisted for as long as there have been DoCs. To grasp the magnitude of the inductive risk, one could imagine that our ability to detect humanity was similarly susceptible to error, and 4 in 10 humans were thought to be nonhuman and were treated accordingly. We might treat them as we do other animals and have them for dinner (no invitation required). That would be a rather dreadful state of affairs, epistemically and ethically.

We can, however, safely say that consciousness is *sufficient* for personhood. Again, we are only speaking of humans for now, but we could just as easily extend this to all conscious entities. There will still be marginal cases that we'll miss, but since we are not ruling out their personhood, not calling them dead, and not making claims about whether they matter morally or can be eaten, the risks of being wrong are minimized. Indeed, one of the benefits of saying that possibly unconscious humans are still persons is that we can coherently make morally informed decisions *on their behalf*. For if we say, on the other hand, that an unconscious human does not matter—is no more than a slab of meat—then we really have no moral reasons to think about their welfare, what might benefit them, and what they would want us to do under the present circumstances. Those are considerations we owe only to persons.

But suppose a reliable, accurate way of determining that someone is conscious (or unconscious) comes along. And suppose also that our ability to predict whether someone with a brain injury will regain consciousness becomes very reliable. To be clear, I doubt very much that either of these innovations will come to pass any time soon, but they are not inconceivable. In other words, suppose the epistemic hurdles can be overcome, and we no longer have to worry about the inductive risks. Should we then accept the Consciousness Criterion? I think not, for the other reasons discussed above.

If TFAHs are persons *only* if they possess X, then whatever X may be, X cannot be consciousness. The Consciousness Criterion is rejected as a *necessary* criterion of being a person or having moral status. I don't think there are any defensible necessary criteria for personhood.

7.6 Pluralism about Persons

My main aim in this chapter is to critique the Consciousness Criterion as a criterion for moral status or personhood, rather than to offer a positive account of moral status or personhood. Efforts to reduce moral status to nonmoral properties like consciousness,

or rationality, or species membership, or what have you don't enhance our moral understanding of what is owed by whom and to
whom, and why. These efforts either make an inferential leap from
nonmoral property X to moral property Y and then to moral status,
or they leap directly from X to moral status. Those leaps don't get
us anywhere useful. The arguments are of questionable soundness,
with premises (e.g., all and only moral agents are persons) that are
not true by necessity or by definition.

The moral status project, that is, the project of trying to define
moral status and who has it, has two aims. One aim is inclusive—
the goal is to define moral status such that those currently outside
the margins can be brought in where they belong. This has been the
project of many, like Regan, who wish to bring some nonhuman
animals inside the moral status circle. The other aim is exclusive
and seeks to define who belongs outside the margins, including
some who are currently inside, or near the margins. This, I think,
is the aim of many who have concluded that unconscious or minimally conscious humans, or humans with intellectual or cognitive
impairments, don't qualify for moral status or personhood. One
project expands the margins, and one contracts them. It's the latter
project that is morally concerning and risky. There is little harm in
treating someone who doesn't matter morally as if they do. Maybe
lobsters don't have moral status, but it harms no one and wrongs
no one (including the lobsters) if I don't eat lobsters on the chance
that they prefer not to be eaten.[21] There is grave potential harm in

---

[21] According to Rachels,

> The concept of moral standing was introduced by philosophers in the 1970s
> to deal with a number of issues that had arisen, such as the treatment of an-
> imals, but also abortion, euthanasia, and the environment. Philosophers
> thought they could make progress in these areas by establishing the moral
> standing of animals, fetuses, comatose persons, trees, and so on. (Rachels
> 2004, 164)

Someone might well object here that it *does* matter whether some entities are mistakenly
thought to have moral status or to be persons. The anti-abortion position that embryos
and fetuses are persons with rights, including a right to life, is one such case. There is no
question that a human embryo or fetus is a living human organism, but that biological

excluding someone and treating them like some *thing*. As moral
agents, we will have failed in our moral obligations to that person,
and we will have treated them wrongly and unjustly and caused
them harm. Having made such mistakes many times in human history, we should be exceedingly careful to avoid them.

The problem with both moral status projects is that they mistakenly treat the resolution of the moral status/personhood question
as if it is the end of moral inquiry rather than the *beginning* of it.
Answering the question *Is Z a person?* in the affirmative *or* the negative only leads to a multitude of further questions about how they
must be treated, what, if anything, is owed to them, and by whom.
For example, if we conclude that dogs are not persons, we must still
decide how dogs must be treated. (My dog Lulu has some thoughts
on the subject of cookies.) If we agreed that individuals in the VS/
UWS are actually dead as persons, we wouldn't just pop them in the
ground while they're still breathing.

That said, although I don't think the concept of moral status or
personhood is especially useful or informative concerning what is
ethically permissible, in the spirit of demonstrating what an *inclusive* conception of personhood might look like, I suggest the following. There are a lot of candidates for *sufficient* properties for
personhood, or for mattering morally. By that I mean, there are a
lot of ways to be a person such that it matters what moral agents do

fact is not conclusive concerning (a) whether it has a right to life, and (b) whether another human being with rights is morally required to sustain its life. The bioethics literature on abortion is voluminous, and I'll not rehearse it more here, but I don't think
invoking fetal moral status has advanced the debate for either side. Instead, it has rather
obscured the importance of the autonomy and bodily sovereignty of pregnant persons.
Someone might argue, still, that there is harm in treating unconscious humans as persons. Gillett argued that it is a mistake to think unconscious humans warrant ethical
concern, and the view is common that it is a consequential mistake to treat unconscious
humans as if they are persons when they are not. I don't think these concerns are best
addressed by attempts to resolve the matter of the qualifications for moral status or
personhood either. The focus on personhood in both these domains has treated moral
status or personhood as if it were the *end* of moral inquiry, rather than the *beginning*.
That is a mistake.

to you and for you. Consciousness is one of them. Being conscious is *enough* to matter morally.

And so is *being human*. Tangwa, commenting on the differences between Western and African conceptions of personhood, noted that

> If the African perception of a person differs from the Western perception, this is not because it does not recognize the various developmental stages of a human being or qualitative differences based on the degree of attainment of positive human attributes or capacities, but rather because it does not draw from these facts the same conclusions as are drawn in Western ethical theory. In particular, the differences between, say, [an intellectually disabled] individual or an infant and a fully self-conscious, mature, rational, and free individual do not entail, in the African perception, that such a being falls outside the "inner sanctum of secular morality" and can or should thus be treated with less moral consideration. (2000, 42)

Tangwa translated the phrase *wir dzë wir*, which in his natal language Lamnso' means "A human being is a human being is a human being, simply by being a human being," which amounts to the belief that moral consideration is due to all humans regardless of their individual characteristics.

Being a member of the species *H. sapiens* is sufficient for personhood, which has two salutary effects. It includes under the protection of personhood all humans, regardless of their age, capacities, or brain function—there are no ethical, epistemic, or metaphysical puzzles about which humans qualify—and it does not exclude other species, or nonhuman entities, from being persons, just in case any are. (I suspect many are.)

Membership in a community of persons is another contender for a criterion of personhood. It is reflected in the traditional Zulu saying, "A person is a person through other people" (Eze 2016,

94). Similarly, the Ubuntu view of personhood can be stated as, "I am because we are." Both express the idea that personhood comes about through participation in the social life of a community of other persons—one is a person because one belongs to a community of persons. This is not a mere tautology, but recognizes the important interconnectedness of persons:

> Persons do not exist as independent islands, floating free of each other—and this is true for all of us. We are cooperative, interconnected beings who depend on the love, support, mutual recognition, purpose, and instruction we receive from each other (although the degree and forms of interdependency vary across individuals and over the course of our lifetimes). Individuals are persons by virtue of being embedded in webs of intersubjective and responsive relationships; our individual capacities emerge only because others nurture us as infants, teach us as toddlers, and cooperate with us as adults. And, here is the heart of the matter, this is true for all of us, equally. . . .
>
> Individuals with cognitive disabilities are no different in this respect. Neither are infants, toddlers, children, adolescents, or persons with mental illness or advanced dementia. They may lack some capacities of typical adults, and the moral duties and citizenship responsibilities that accompany them. Nonetheless, all of them are fully embedded in the web of interpersonal relationships in which personhood is realized. (Andrews et al. 2019)

This way of being a person may sound circular, or precarious. *A person is a person because they belong to a community of persons* seems to leave us hanging as to the entry point, but also to the potential exits (or forced exits). But it doesn't. We are all born into communities of at least a few persons, and none of us could survive the neonatal period if we were not. It's not easy to be excluded, either. Even Romulus and Remus, although abandoned at birth, condemned to die, nursed by a she-wolf, and fed by a woodpecker, were eventually reabsorbed into the human community of persons into which they were born.

There is something else that's important about belonging to a community of persons. What moral agents do to, and for, one member of the community matters to the others, and so the direct duties of moral agents multiply. As discussed above, we can harm psychologically complex persons by harming those they care about. I don't mean here that infanticide only harms the parents and not the infant, or that shooting a dog only harms the dog's human and not the dog. I mean that moral agents have duties to the dog and the dog's human and to the infant and the parents. Their burdens are many.

We might name or list any number of the other capacities that have been mentioned above as sufficient for personhood: autonomy, rationality, being a moral agent. Any of them is enough. It's important that our criteria be enduring, nonfluctuating, and epistemically robust, and one way to achieve that, given the vicissitudes of life, is to be pluralist about the sufficient conditions for personhood. There is more than one door into personhood. So long as our criteria are sufficient but not necessary, we won't push anyone outside the margins when they have a right to be inside, and the risk of mistakenly including someone who doesn't belong is minor and worth taking. In its favor, the inductive risks of the inclusive moral status project are fewer and smaller than those of the exclusionary project. If we must engage in a moral status project, it is better—epistemically and ethically—that we engage in the inclusive one.

8

Disorders of Consciousness and the Disability Critique

Brain injuries can result in short-term, long-term, and chronic disability. Disorders of consciousness (DoCs) may count as disabilities, although they are not paradigmatic disabilities like mobility or sensory disabilities. The prevention of disability and DoCs following brain injury motivates some withdrawals of life-sustaining treatment (LST) in neurointensive care. Withdrawals of LST in chronic DoCs, and specifically withdrawal of artificial nutrition and hydration (ANH), are controversial among some disability activists and scholars. The entanglement of questions, concerns, fears, and uncertainties related to brain injuries, DoCs, and disabilities is complex, and may not be amenable to disentangling. But I'll try.

8.1 Impairment and Disability

The terms *impairment* and *disability* are not used interchangeably among disability scholars and disabled persons.[1] *Impairment* is frequently used to refer to conditions of the body that depart from

---

[1] Two points of note: First, I use the term *disabled person(s)* preferentially in this book. Both *disabled persons* and *persons with disabilities* are terms that involve ideological commitments and cannot be viewed as neutral or bias-free. Importantly, some disabled persons, including some members of the Deaf and autism communities, reject "person-first" language. Second, this chapter does not provide an overview of theories of disability. Neither does it focus on the metaphysics of disability, as interesting as that is. That work has been capably done elsewhere (see, for example, Sherry 2013; Albrecht, Seelman, and Bury 2001; and Barnes 2016).

what is considered typical (or "normal"), whereas *disability* often refers to the effects of social structures or reactions to impairments, such as discrimination (ableism), marginalization, oppression, and exclusion. In this way, disability can be viewed as "socially constructed"—what makes a difference of the body disabling is the way that it is perceived by society, or the way society is structured to exclude or marginalize those with physical differences (Sherry 2013; Shakespeare 2006). According to the social model, disability is contextual, and not all *impaired* people are disabled in the same ways, in the same contexts. On a stronger reading of the social model, impairments in the absence of prejudice would not be significant (Barnes 2016).

According to the social model, what is disabling about impairments is remediable by changing society and institutions, rather than changing disabled persons and their bodies. Disability is caused by injustice, so "fixing" it is a matter of justice.

The social model of disability contrasts with what is referred to as the "medical model" or the "individual model," an essentialist view of disability that situates it solely in individual deficit(s) and views it as "an individual tragedy or misfortune due to genetic or environmental insult" (Reynolds 2017). On the medicalized view, "People with disabilities are assumed to suffer primarily from physical and/or mental abnormalities that medicine can and should treat, cure, or at least prevent" (Wendell 2001). On the medical model, fixing "abnormal" bodies is the remedy for disability.

Critics of the social model point out that it neglects the way impairments really do influence people's lives and can be problems in their own right, even without the influence of social structures and biases. As Barnes has noted, some proponents of the social model appear committed to the idea that in order to say that disability is not bad, "we have to say that disabilities would, in the absence of ableism, not have any bad effects" (Barnes 2016, 27). Barnes has rejected as implausible that

All, or at least the most substantial, bad effects of disability are socially mediated. . . . At least for many disabilities, there would be things about them that were difficult or unpleasant even in an ideal society. And while many people value and enjoy being disabled, not everyone values and enjoys being disabled. (2016, 78)

The experience of chronic pain, or degenerative/progressive conditions that can cause premature death, are disabling in ways that cannot be explained in wholly sociopolitical terms (Shakespeare 2006). As Wendell pointed out, "Some unhealthy disabled people, as well as some healthy people with disabilities, experience physical or psychological burdens that no amount of social justice can eliminate" (Wendell 2001).

8.2 Are Patients with DoCs Disabled?

DoCs can involve simultaneously various physical, motor, sensory, communication, and cognitive impairments. One way in which they differ from paradigmatic forms of disability like sensory or mobility impairments is that little that is disabling about DoCs can be defined as socially constructed. That affected individuals cannot communicate or participate in social life and employment is a result of the impairments and incapacities caused by injury to their brains. Impairments of consciousness involve a number of what Tom Shakespeare (2006) has called "intrinsic limitations" that are not remediable through accommodation.[2] While persons with acute or chronic brain injuries can be both impaired and socially disabled, and there is no doubt that persons with DoCs are also

---

[2] There have been some experimental efforts to establish communication with DoC patients, using imaging modalities like functional magnetic resonance imaging (fMRI). Brain–computer interfaces are hypothetical possibilities. To date, the communication that has been possible has been quite limited, owing in part to the cumbersome and time-consuming technology required.

persons with brain injuries, DoCs may well be special cases where there is an incomplete overlap with the concerns of disability rights advocates and scholars. DoCs are disabling in ways that are not well explained by the social model.

However, medical resources like rehabilitation for persons with neurological injuries are difficult to access. These services are scarce, expensive, and not geographically or financially accessible to many. The reasons for this are at least partly explained by priorities in the distribution of social and healthcare resources. The expense of rehabilitation and the devaluation of disabled persons, especially those who are less visible, are certainly factors. Specialized neurorehabilitation has been shown to improve functioning and the recovery of consciousness for some DoC patients (Giacino et al. 2018), so the lack of availability and the financial inaccessibility of neurorehabilitation can be *disabling* in the ways described by the social model—the result of unjust discrimination and marginalization. To put it in perspective, consider the wide accessibility of treatment and rehabilitation for sport-related physical injuries like ACL tears or tennis elbow, and the sizable expenditure in healthcare resources for both professional athletes and weekend warriors. We could easily explain the social and financial neglect of persons with DoCs, their marginalization, and invisibility, as discriminatory, and the consequence of a more widespread and long-standing neglect of disabled people *as people*, let alone as people with sometimes complex and specialized resource needs.[3]

8.3 Withdrawing LST and DoCs: The Disability Rights Critique

Some members of disability communities and activist organizations have strenuously objected to the withdrawal of LST, specifically

---

[3] Joseph Fins and Megan Wright, for example, have characterized the neglect of American DoC patients as violations of the Americans with Disabilities Act (Fins and Wright 2018; Fins 2015).

ANH, from persons in the vegetative state/unresponsive wakeful-ness syndrome (VS/UWS). Not Dead Yet successfully protested for state intervention when Terri Schiavo's surrogate, her husband Michael Schiavo, sought to have her feeding tube removed in 2005 (Johnson 2005). Harriet McBryde Johnson argued that Schiavo's feeding tube counted as "adaptive equipment" (which it surely is for many disabled persons) and not medical treatment that a patient's surrogate could refuse on their behalf. Schiavo had been diagnosed in a VS/UWS for 15 years and was certainly neither legally dead nor terminally ill.[4] Withdrawing ANH, depending on how one views it, was intended either to hasten her death by starvation or to not arti-ficially prolong a life she would not have wanted to live. Either way of describing it is tendentious. In the view of some activists, Schiavo was a disabled person subjected to life-threatening anti-disability discrimination, a victim of the "better dead than disabled" bias (Johnson 2006).

To many disabled persons, Schiavo's fate could have been their own. Indeed, that is precisely what was expressed in an amicus brief filed in *Bush v. Schiavo*:

> [A] close examination of the issues shows that Schiavo's fate is intertwined with that of many people with disabilities who must rely on surrogates. If the legal standard of proof in cases involving termination of life support is watered down to the point where Ms. Schiavo's "quality of life"—as determined by others—justifies her death, then one cannot distinguish Ms. Schiavo from any-one else who is "incompetent," including thousands who cannot speak due to developmental or physical disabilities. It is naïve to believe such attitudes would not be used to justify the death of

---

[4] Terri Schiavo's CT scans showed that much of her brain tissue had atrophied, with significant hydrocephalus ex vacuo, in which cerebrospinal fluid fills the cavity left by ventricular atrophy. In other words, much of her brain was not only nonfunctioning, but also no longer there.

people with severe disabilities if the opportunity arose. (Rahdert et al. 2004)

8.3.1 Denial of Treatment or Treatment Refusal?

The amicus brief equates the withdrawal of ANH in Schiavo's case as a *denial* of medical treatment to a disabled person rather than a *refusal* of unwanted medical treatment, noting that in the United States, "withholding of medical treatment based on disability has a long, pervasive and tragic history" (Rahdert et al. 2004). The amici thus sought to draw a bright line between a patient's own "firm and settled commitment" to refuse or terminate life support and a surrogate's substituted judgments about patient preferences or best interests. The distinction between denial of treatment and refusal of treatment pits against each other two important patient rights: the right to refuse treatment and the right to life.

Patients with decisional capacity have long had an unconditional right to refuse unwanted medical treatment, a right undergirded by the rights of privacy, bodily integrity, and respect for individual autonomy. Treatment without consent is trespass and assault, per Justice Benjamin Cardozo:

> Every human being of adult years and sound mind has a right to determine what shall be done with his own body; and a surgeon who performs an operation without his patient's consent, commits an assault, for which he is liable in damages. . . . This is true except in cases of emergency where the patient is unconscious and where it is necessary to operate before consent can be obtained. (*Schloendorff v. New York Hospital* 1914)

The right to refuse covers both refusals of treatment by competent persons and advance decisions made by formerly competent patients. While supporters of the "right to die" may cast the right to medical aid in dying (MAiD) as similarly grounded in autonomy, it is not straightforwardly so. MAiD, unlike treatment refusal, asserts a positive right to a medical intervention. That both MAiD and withdrawing LST can result in the death of a patient does not mean they are grounded in the same rights or principles. Some in the disabled community see the right to life of disabled persons, and especially those who are incapacitated, as in conflict with the right to die, and they view endorsement of a right to die or to MAiD as a threat to disabled persons. The fear, reasonably based on a history of medical neglect, is that paternalistic views about the badness of life with disability will lead to involuntary euthanasia of disabled persons. Andrew Batavia argued against characterizing disabled persons as vulnerable and oppressed (Batavia 2001), and viewed efforts to protect disabled persons from "assisted dying" as unjustifiably paternalistic and at odds with autonomy and self-determination. He argued that "people with disabilities should be allowed to make all decisions that affect their lives, including the decision to end their lives with or without assistance" (Batavia 2003). To the extent that the right to refuse treatment and the right to die are viewed strictly as autonomy-based rights, those rights are not available to those who have never been autonomous or legally competent. Neither can their surrogates claim such rights on their behalf. This creates a dual standard that could potentially cause harm to some persons with developmental or cognitive disabilities, like Sheila Pouliot.

Alicia Ouellette has criticized what she calls the "new activists" in the disability rights movement who have taken a strong right-to-life stance—which Ouellette has characterized as "perniciously paternalistic"—concerning the withdrawal of feeding tubes from incapacitated patients like Schiavo (Ouellette 2006). Ouellette's concern is that limiting the ability of surrogates to make decisions to withdraw LST in order to protect disabled persons will paternalistically endanger *all* incapacitated persons by forcing treatment on those who cannot refuse it. Ironically, it is also paternalism—of surrogates and medical staff—that is the target of disabled persons in this fight. They see judgments about their best interests and quality of life used as justifications for withdrawing treatment and ending their lives. Echoing the statement in the amicus brief is this pointed expression from a joint statement by several disability rights organizations:

> If the legal standard in cases involving termination of life support is reduced to the point where Ms. Schindler-Schiavo's 'quality of life'—as determined by others—justifies her death by starvation, then what protections exist for the thousands of us who cannot speak due to disabilities? (ADA Watch et al. 2003)

The proposed solution to this threat is to prevent anyone— medical staff, family member, legal guardian, or surrogate—from choosing to end LST for patients who lack decisional capacity, absent clear and convincing evidence of the patients' wishes. But it is disconcerting at best to call that *protection* in circumstances where treatment prolongs suffering at the end of life, or when the affected individual would prefer to have treatment withdrawn. It potentially leads to something akin to patients "rotting with their rights on," protected in ways that may run counter to their interests or desires.[5]

Squaring protection of vulnerable persons with autonomy can be a considerable challenge. For persons who are legally competent and have decisional capacity, it is not paternalistic to protect their right and ability to make their own decisions about medical treatment. Indeed, this is what disabled persons have long fought for: to not have their self-determination usurped by others to limit

---

[5] The memorable phrase "rotting with their rights on" originated in the 1970s in considerations of treatment *refusals* by hospitalized psychiatric patients (Appelbaum and Gutheil 1979). The concern was that patients who refused medical treatment in contexts where they were not free to leave would essentially be left to rot, untreated, but with their autonomy/bodily integrity rights intact. This concern is also apt in contexts where a patient's condition is such that continued treatment prolongs life but may lead to iatrogenic suffering, as in the case of Sheila Pouliot (*Blouin v. Spitzer* 2002; Ouellette 2004). Descriptions of Ms. Pouliot's unfortunate and painful condition at the end of life give almost literal meaning to "rotting with their rights on."

their medical treatment or to terminate their lives against their will. When a person has prospectively made those choices in anticipation of future need, such as in an advance directive, honoring their choices respects their autonomy, even when they are no longer able to exercise that autonomy in the present. The *Schiavo* amici quoted the *Cruzan* decision as supporting the incapacitated patient's right to treatment limitations or terminations based solely on "clear and convincing evidence" of "a *firm* and *settled commitment* to the termination of life supports under the circumstances" (Rahdert et al. 2004). Yet some disability scholars express doubts about the ability of non-disabled individuals, or families, to make informed decisions about the prospect of a future life with a disability:

> From the standpoint of disability rights, the most serious flaw of advance directives is that asserted by bioethicists Dresser and Robertson (1989), who criticize the "orthodox" reliance on any advance statement of preferences. People who are not living as individuals with disabilities and cannot imagine that their lives as disabled would be satisfying make such advance statements to them. . . . Dresser and Robertson urge that nondisabled people acknowledge the value of disabled life and evaluate treatment decision making from the perspective of the now disabled individual. (Asch 2001, 310)

Rebecca Dresser and John Robertson criticized the "orthodox approach":

> It is difficult, if not impossible, for competent individuals to predict their interests in future treatment situations when they are incompetent because their needs and interests will have so radically changed. (1989, 236)

They cited as an "error" the assumption that expressed or inferred prior choices accurately indicate an incompetent individual's current interests. Dresser and Robertson argued that honoring advance directives involves a normative judgment that it is more important to give persons presumed control against unwanted *overtreatment* than it is to prevent mistakes of *undertreatment*. That is, it is a judgment that it is more important to protect autonomy-based treatment refusals than to protect persons from preventable deaths.

> The security gained in empowering persons to control their medical future in this way is not cost-free. The cost—too often overlooked—is that adherence to the directive will lead to the death of incompetent patients who retain significant interests in continued life. (1989, 237)

Dresser and Robertson were concerned that the conceptual confusions contained in the "orthodox approach" to honoring advance directives "threatens to harm conscious incompetent patients" (Dresser and Robertson 1989, 236), and in particular, "victims of stroke, senility, Alzheimer's disease, and other illnesses" (234). They specifically exempt *unconscious* patients from the same analysis, noting (consistent with another orthodox view) that they lack "significant interests in prolonged life" and "cannot experience any benefit from continued life" (Dresser and Robertson 1989, 241–242). Of the minimally conscious, they noted,

> Although some will argue that any minimally conscious human being has a significant stake in being maintained, it is difficult to see how life without greater awareness of self and others can confer a genuine benefit on these patients. Families who take this position and request non-treatment would not therefore be violating the right to life of such patients. (242)

For minimally conscious patients who can experience pains and pleasures, it is possible that life *might* be a continued benefit, but also possible that it is not. While Dresser and Robertson placed these individuals in the same category as unconscious patients, U.S. courts have been hesitant to do the same, instead erring on the side of caution, continued life, and continued LST (Johnson 2011; Johnson and Cerminara 2020).[6] The analysis of advance directives by Dresser and Robertson, then, partially but not wholly supports the concerns of disability advocates about undertreatment and withdrawal of LST from disabled persons. In the case of Terri Schiavo, diagnosed as unconscious for more than a decade, Dresser and Robertson would not find fault in her surrogate's decision to withdraw LST, nor would we find in their analysis wholesale support for advance directives that accord with the *Cruzan* standard of providing "clear and convincing evidence," because of what they describe as the

> ultimate indeterminacy of the fiction of treating the incompetent patient as a self-determining individual. While the predominant danger of the orthodox approach is undertreatment, it also poses a risk that unjustified overtreatment will occur whenever the courts impose a strict standard for inferring the patient's choice if competent. In that case, medical zeal and rigid concern with right to life values may override patient and other interests. (1989, 240)

8.3.2 Between a Rock and a Hard Place Again: Paternalism v. Paternalism

During the protracted legal battle over the withdrawal of Terri Schiavo's feeding tube, the trial court found that previous

---

[6] Other jurisdictions treat MCS patients much the same as VS/UWS patients. In the United Kingdom, for example, where treatment withdrawals require court approvals, the courts generally permit withdrawal for MCS patients, as well as many other patients, following a "best interests" standard. The M case, discussed in chapter 6, is a notable exception.

expressions concerning LST made by Terri Schiavo satisfied the standard of "clear and convincing evidence."

> Statements which Terri Schiavo made which do support the relief sought by her surrogate (Petitioner/Guardian) include statements to him prompted by her grandmother being in intensive care that if she was ever a burden she would not want to live like that. Additionally, statements made to Michael Schiavo which were prompted by something on television regarding people on life support that she would not want to life [sic] like that also reflect her intention in this particular situation. Also statements she made in the presence of Scott Schiavo at the funeral luncheon for his grandmother that "if I ever go like that just let me go. Don't leave me there. I don't want to be kept alive on a machine." And to Joan Schiavo following a television movie in which a man following an accident was in a coma to the effect that she wanted it stated in her will that she would want the tubes and everything taken out if that ever happened to her are likewise reflective of this intent. (Judge George Greer in *In re: Schiavo* 2000)

The court specifically rejected statements reportedly made by Schiavo when she was a child, concerning the Karen Ann Quinlan case. Schiavo's statements, as reported by her family members, were remarkably similar—sometimes word for word—to statements made by Robert Wendland, including "just let me go." In Wendland's case, because he was in the minimally conscious state (MCS) and not a persistent vegetative state (PVS), they were discounted.

The disability rights organizations that opposed withdrawing ANH from Schiavo drew parallels between disabled persons, particularly those with cognitive disabilities, and those with DoCs:

[Terri Schiavo] has a severe brain injury, yet has not undergone the rehabilitation that is typically given to people with this type of disability.[7] People with severe cognitive disabilities are devalued as lives not worth living. In truth, the lives of all of us with severe disabilities are often considered expendable. This is why we are speaking out.

Americans who have disabilities—cognitive disabilities like Ms. Schindler-Schiavo—have rights. Congress decided that in 1990 when it passed the Americans with Disabilities Act. Yet most of society does not consider that Terri Schindler-Schiavo has any rights other than the right to die. We believe she has a right to therapy and support; we believe the Americans with Disabilities Act requires that.

The fear of disability and the resulting bigotry adhered to by most non-disabled Americans is often cited by people with disabilities as one of the most difficult barriers to overcome. In a recent column, Bill Press stated, "I wouldn't want to live like that, would you?" We respond: "like what?" Terri Schindler-Schiavo is characterized as " . . . a brain-damaged woman who has been kept alive artificially." Meant to signal horror, the concept has no real meaning to us who live by "artificial" means. (ADA Watch et al. 2003)

Whereas Karen Ann Quinlan's case first brought to public attention the persistent VS and helped launch the right-to-die movement, in Schiavo disability rights activists found a highly visible embodiment of the vulnerability, marginalization, erasure, and threat to life that many disabled persons fear and experience. Schiavo's husband and guardian, Michael Schiavo, came to

---

[7] The statement that Schiavo did not receive rehabilitation is incorrect. She did receive rehabilitative therapy for a number of years, including treatment with an experimental thalamic stimulator, a brain implant that can be seen in the CT scans of her brain (Cerminara and Goodman 2020). It is also not true that people with severe brain injuries typically have access to specialized neurorehabilitation, although they should.

represent the untrustworthy surrogate, "on a quest to remove his wife's source of nourishment" and to starve her to death (ADA Watch et al. 2003).

There is inherent and likely unresolvable tension in the various positions staked out in this debate. The autonomy and right of self-determination of disabled persons to make their own medical decisions is decidedly in tension with the paternalism of requiring an exceptionally strict standard for what counts as "clear and convincing" evidence of prior wishes for incapacitated patients (a standard that many written advance directives would fail to satisfy, but which was met in Schiavo's case). Rejecting as uninformed the advance directives made by formerly competent, non-disabled persons just in case they become disabled and incompetent is similarly paternalistic. As Barnes argued, it is

> plausible that some people wouldn't like being disabled even in an ideal society. And I think such preferences should be listened to and respected—not dismissed as implicitly ableist or obviously caused by social prejudice—just as the preferences of those who value disability should be listened to and respected. (2016, 78)

Also paternalistic is restricting surrogates and families from making decisions to limit treatment, even when, in good faith, they attempt to make those decisions in accordance with the values and interests of the disabled patient in mind. Families do also seek to continue medical treatment that some medical staff view as pointless or harmful, because doing so aligns with their own and the patient's values. Restrictions that limit surrogates thus attempt to square using paternalism to protect against paternalism by paternalistically protecting disabled persons from the misguided paternalism of surrogates and medical staff.

8.4 Who Has the Epistemic Authority to Speak for DoC Patients?

Fricker identified *testimonial injustice* as a distinct form of *epistemic injustice* in which prejudicial stereotypes distort credibility judgments. This kind of injustice has multiple effects. It can obviously act as an obstacle to truth and the circulation of true beliefs and knowledge. More importantly, great injustices might be experienced by speakers who are undermined or ignored because of the unjust deficit of credibility they are granted. As Fricker noted, it can be dangerously dehumanizing.

> We are long familiar with the idea, played out by the history of philosophy in many variations, that our rationality is what lends humanity its distinctive value. No wonder, then, that being insulted, undermined, or otherwise wronged in one's capacity as a giver of knowledge is something that can cut deep. No wonder too that in contexts of oppression the powerful will be sure to undermine the powerless in just that capacity, for it provides a direct route to undermining them in their very humanity. (2007, 44)

In chapter 4 I discuss inferences about the quality of life of disabled people, and how value judgments about disability add uncertainty and pessimism to prognosis. Epistemic privilege or authority is generally granted to non-disabled persons to make choices for *themselves* based on their judgments about whether they would value life with a disability. Their authority is based not on their knowledge about disability—which may be scant—but rather their self-knowledge concerning their own values and preferences. Medical staff and surrogates have long enjoyed similar epistemic privilege, mostly without justification. Fricker would call that a "credibility excess," and it too is a form of epistemic injustice. (Individuals might be wrong about their own preferences and values, or they might be mistaken about what their lives would be like with a disability, but I don't think they do injustice to themselves by granting themselves an excess of credibility, or that others unjustly grant them excess credibility. Credibility excess becomes unjust when there is an unwarranted credibility deficit for some other knower.) Disabled persons are right to claim epistemic privilege and authority for themselves, and to have the same rights of autonomy and self-determination, and the right to be respected as knowers, as anyone else.

Prejudicial attitudes that track people across all the domains of their lives and result in systematic injustice are, as Fricker noted, forms of "identity prejudice," and identity prejudice influences the credibility of speakers and knowers (Fricker 2007, 28). The undermining of the credibility of disabled persons to speak for and about themselves, and their experiences of disability, is the result of identity prejudice, and an example of testimonial injustice. In this light, we can view the so-called disability paradox—the idea that it is a mystery that disabled persons have better quality of life than non-disabled persons think is possible—as an example of epistemic, testimonial injustice.

But. Autonomy rights belong to individuals. Epistemic privilege, the right to be listened to with respect and be treated as an authority, also rightly belongs to individuals, those in a position to have authority and knowledge, rather than to those who can merely speculate or imagine (or who have credibility in other spheres). Disabled persons are right to claim epistemic privilege and authority where they have knowledge, experience, and expertise. But we might well ask if they have that knowledge, experience, and expertise concerning life with a DoC.

There have been only a handful of published first-person accounts of patients who emerged from DoCs, and who were treated as though they were still unconscious (that is, misdiagnosed patients; see Tavalaro and Tayson 1997; Pistorius 2013; Lunau 2015; Macniven et al. 2003; Wilson, Gracey, and Bainbridge 2001). It is possible (perhaps likely) that there is considerable overlap in the experiences of other persons with brain injuries and those in the MCS or those who have emerged from the MCS, and to that extent, we might well look to others with brain injuries to inform us. But given the diversity of disability and experience, and because disabled persons are *individuals*, not every disabled person can speak for every other disabled person. Wheelchair users may not be well-situated to speak about those with cognitive and developmental disabilities. Those with hidden disabilities may not experience the same forms and expressions of discrimination, or the same socially constructed disabilities, experienced by others. Women, queer, and BIPOC disabled persons experience different biases and manifestations of discrimination and bigotry at the intersections of disability, race, and gender (Bailey and Mobley 2019; National Disability Alliance Steering Committee 2020). The point is not that disabled persons have no authority or credibility to speak about other disabled persons, or persons with different disabilities. The point is that there is the same diversity among disabled persons— diversity of experiences, preferences, values—that there is among people in general, and so it cannot be assumed that just *any* disabled person is best situated to have epistemic access to the subjective experiences of any other disabled person. To think that all disabled persons are alike is as flattening, erasing, and damaging as to think that all women, or all Indigenous persons, or all queer persons, are alike.

If we accept that non-disabled persons lack the epistemic authority to speak *for* disabled persons, we ought, for the same reasons, doubt that paradigmatically disabled persons can speak *for* those with DoCs. That leaves us with three possibilities. Where a person made their wishes known in an advance directive or by informing a healthcare proxy, we can be guided by their expressed preferences, accepting the possibility that their past preferences may have been imperfectly informed. Where they did not, or where they were never capable of doing so, we can rely on families and surrogates to make decisions about treatment and treatment limitations. Or we can protect disabled persons from potentially misguided surrogate decisions by restricting the authority of surrogates to make some, or any, decisions. All options carry the risk that decisions made on behalf of these patients will not align with their current interests or preferences, if they have any. Asch described the motivation for restricting surrogate decision-making or control over disabled persons who lack the capacity or authority to decide for themselves:

> For situations in which families typically are expected to act on behalf of those who cannot make their wishes known, disability rights adherents remain skeptical about the good faith of much purported ·family decision-making. Fearful of covert or overt bias against a now-disabled or lifelong-disabled family member who never provided an advance directive, and convinced that people without disabilities doubt the value of life with an impairment, those holding a disability rights perspective would look to governments and courts to protect the interests of vulnerable individuals and would seek all methods to improve the chances that disabled people themselves will participate in these decisions. It is crucial for anyone seeking to advance the dignity and worth of people with all disabilities to promote their own participation in life-and-death decisions and to circumscribe family decision making on behalf of those who have less than full legal authority to make their own decisions. (2001, 311)

It is not clear that anyone—including other disabled persons—can meaningfully speak for DoC patients in a way that is *better* than speaking to the values, preferences, and interests they had in the past. DoC patients have interests that carry over from their life before, and some may have an interest in continued life, while others may not. If they have any current interests, they are not accessible or comprehensible to those with unimpaired consciousness, which complicates comparisons to disabled persons who uncontroversially do have current interests, preferences, and desires.

In recognizing the motive behind the disability community's activism in the Schiavo case, Asch acknowledged that the alignment of interests was imperfect, but not nonexistent.

> Schiavo's supporters in the disability community were almost certainly mistaken about her potential for interaction or responsiveness, and they may have done damage to their efforts to join with others seeking to reform treatment of disabled or dying people. Yet the apprehension in the disability community, apprehension about societal indifference and neglect, is more understandable after reviewing a few of the many instances in which law, medicine, bioethics, and government programs failed to help traumatically disabled patients discover the financial, technological, social, and psychological resources that could sustain them and provide the opportunity for rewarding life. When people with relatively intact cognitive and emotional capacities are neglected, neglect is even more likely for those with greatly diminished cognitive and emotional function. (2005, S34)

The interests of right-to-die activists and of disability activists and scholars *can* align when it comes to maximizing and ensuring the self-determination and autonomy of patients in their interactions with medicine—both groups should, and do, oppose testimonial injustice in medicine and health law and policy. Their common cause is broken, however, by the way the former often view, talk about, and weaponize disability and quality of life in ways that undermine the autonomy and self-determination of disabled persons. In cases like Schiavo's, some disability activists have thus moved to the right-to-life side of the debate, leaving them on the uncomfortable horns of a dilemma, adopting paternalistic solutions to the problem of threatened autonomy. Other disability scholars, like Batavia, reject that paternalism and the implication that disabled persons are vulnerable victims, easily pressured into ending their lives.

The disability-rights movement has been successful in securing a broad array of rights for people with disabilities, and these rights are based in large part on the recognition of their autonomy. People with disabilities have the right to be free of involuntary sterilization, to raise children, to be educated in public schools, to use public transportation, and to have access to places of public accommodation. We believe that competent persons with disabilities, even in the oppressive circumstances of many institutions, are capable of autonomy. Most disabled persons do not consider themselves vulnerable or oppressed and want to make the decisions that fundamentally affect their lives. (1997)

When the debate concerns persons like Terri Schiavo, who are not paradigmatically disabled, who are not autonomous, and who cannot exercise self-determination in the present, the right-to-life alliance may not be one that can be maintained without risking the autonomy of all disabled persons and subjecting them to unjustifiable paternalism. But, as Not Dead Yet president Diane Coleman has pointed out, disabled persons frequently find themselves caught between two conflicting and damaging positions, and excluded from policymaking that *concerns* them, but is carried on *without* them:

The far right wants to kill us slowly and painfully by cutting the things we need to live, health care, public housing and transportation, etc. The far left wants to kill us quickly and call it compassion, while also saving money for others perhaps deemed more worthy. (Quoted in Asch 2005, S35)

Upholding the testimonial credibility of disabled persons requires that we give credence to those individual persons whose views (past or present) about their own fates may be influenced more by identity prejudice than is comfortable or preferable. This is a considerable epistemic and ethical dilemma. Avoiding the problem of testimonial injustice requires epistemic humility, a willingness to accept the epistemic authority and credibility of individuals speaking for themselves, even when we think they might be mistaken or ill-informed. This may be especially difficult to accept when the societally dominant view has the potential for dangerous spillover effects for those who are marginalized and have minority views. Dogmatic acceptance of the better-dead-than-disabled view can have dangerous effects for disabled persons if their own testimonial credibility is discounted or denied. But testimonial credibility is not a zero-sum game. There is not less credibility to go around if we are generous with it, even if we give too much credibility where it may not be warranted. Giving testimonial and epistemic credibility to the preferences of non-disabled (or newly disabled) persons does not imply that other disabled persons should have less credibility than others. Indeed, their credibility and authority to speak for themselves is warranted for exactly the same reasons—the subjectivity of individual experience, preferences, and values.

8.5 Upstream Ableism

Ableism or anti-disability bias—whether implicit or explicit— undoubtedly influences upstream treatment withdrawal decisions. Disability that is not compatible with a good and flourishing life is one of the downstream outcomes that upstream action seeks to avoid. It must be acknowledged that not everyone does recover awareness, and of those who do, not everyone recovers all the capacities and abilities that, prior to their injuries, they considered important to a good and flourishing life. Respecting individual autonomy requires that we respect the right of persons to make decisions about their own possible futures, whether those decisions are based on a false sense of hopefulness, or of hopelessness. There is an inherent tension in doing so, but acknowledging and holding that tension demonstrates due deference and epistemic humility, and acknowledges the extent to which there are no one-size-fits-all solutions. One concern when a substantial proportion of deaths in neurointensive care follow withdrawal of LST is that a limited and prejudicial view of possible outcomes has an outsized influence on decisions. When withdrawal of LST is viewed as the solution, the "problems" it solves—a bad or prolonged death, or a bad life, or life with disability—are uncritically viewed as worse, and not worth risking.

While downstream, end-of-life battles over patients (like Terri Schiavo) with DoCs often garner a great deal of public attention and renew long-standing public and bioethical debates about the value of consciousness and life, the many decisions to limit or withdraw treatment that occur upstream, in neurointensive care, are largely hidden from sight. The covert influence of ableism is there, too.

8.5.1 Implicit and Explicit Bias in Decision-Making on Behalf of Brain-Injured Patients

Implicit and explicit bias toward disability and disabled persons on the part of medical staff and surrogates influence upstream decisions, and in particular the upstream conclusion that the patient would be "better off dead." When PVS was named and described in 1972, there was little to be done for patients beyond life-sustaining measures. Half a century later, treatment options remain very limited, but we know that DoCs are far more varied, and prognosis is far less certain. Nonetheless, the nihilistic belief in hopelessness has persisted, expressed by medical staff, bioethicists, by statutes, courts, and individuals.

Faced with uncertainty, surrogates often turn to medical staff when making decisions about treatment and withdrawal of LST. Some surrogates recognize that *prognostic* uncertainty exists— after all, it involves predicting the future—but nonetheless prefer to discuss uncertain prognoses for a number of important reasons, including that

> beliefs that prognostic uncertainty is unavoidable, that physicians are the best and only source for prognostic information, and that discussing prognostic uncertainty leaves room for realistic hope, increases surrogates' trust in the physician, allows surrogates time to prepare to make difficult life support decisions, and to prepare for possible bereavement. (Evans et al. 2009)

Because of the epistemic asymmetries, the vulnerability of surrogates, and their reliance on medical staff, biases among medical staff can have an outsized influence on decision-making. Medical staff who counsel surrogates and families as they make decisions about patients have an epistemic duty to acknowledge the uncertainty, and their own biases and value judgments.

8.5.2 Implicit Bias Among Medical Staff

Whether or not patients have advance directives, hospital-based physicians are less accurate at predicting end-of-life and treatment preferences for patients than are family members, and none of these potential decision makers predicts patient preferences very well (Coppola et al. 2001; Sullivan 2002). Research spanning decades shows that physician values have a strong influence on treatment and nontreatment decisions, despite their incongruence with patient preferences and wishes (Orentlicher 1992). This raises important concerns about the potential for bias in interactions between medical staff and surrogates.

Physicians and other medical staff are biased in ways that are similar to, and similar in degree to, the ways the general population is biased (FitzGerald and Hurst 2017). In particular, they harbor "aversive" biases, in which they explicitly reject a bias (such as racism), but are found to have implicit racial biases when the Implicit Association Test is administered.[8] Thus, while professional and ethical standards in medicine support norms of impartiality and oppose prejudice and bias, medical staff, like everyone else, harbor implicit biases that may conflict with their avowed attitudes and commitments. This is concerning if those biases influence how they treat patients or advise patient surrogates. Indeed, there is clear evidence of a relationship between implicit bias and negative effects on clinical interactions. Numerous studies have found that provider–patient interactions are influenced by bias, and that "some kind of bias was evident in either the diagnosis, the treatment recommendations, the number of questions asked of the patient, the number of tests ordered, or other responses indicating bias against the characteristics of the patient under examination" (FitzGerald and Hurst 2017, 13). The influence of bias cuts across all categories of persons who are frequently subject to discrimination, including BIPOC, LGBTQ+, and disabled persons. The majority of healthcare workers self-report no biases against disabled persons, but implicitly, the overwhelming majority are biased against the disabled and in favor of the non-disabled, exhibiting "aversive ableism" (VanPuymbrouck, Friedman, and Feldner 2020).[9]

> Direct assessments of implicit and explicit attitudes toward people with physical disabilities reveal results similar to those for race: Implicit attitudes show significant bias against people with disabilities while explicit attitudes yield little evidence of prejudice; also, implicit and explicit attitudes are only weakly related.

---

[8] The Implicit Association Test (IAT) is a validated and widely used test of implicit biases. The Disability Attitudes Implicit Association Test (DA-IAT) is a validated instrument for measuring bias against disability and in favor of "ability" (Gould et al. 2019), or what is called "ableism."

[9] The same study found that about 10 percent of healthcare staff were both explicitly and implicitly biased against disabled persons, while only about 2 percent showed little implicit or explicit bias (VanPuymbrouck, Friedman, and Feldner 2020).

These biases occur even among professionals who work directly with people with disabilities. (Dovidio, Pagotto, and Hebl 2011)

The greatest danger of implicit biases is that while they *do* influence behavior at an unconscious level, they are not under rational control or conscious influence, and are thus difficult to identify and overcome. Because they are implicit, and people do not view implicit biases or prejudices as expressions of the attitudes they consciously endorse, they do not try to control or counter them. Importantly, when people are prejudiced in an aversive fashion, "they also often rationalize their prejudice and justify it as not biased" (VanPuymbrouck, Friedman, and Feldner 2020). Thus, we see poor "quality of life" frequently invoked as a reason to limit or withhold treatment for a disabled or potentially disabled patient, as it was in Michael Hickson's case. The results can be deadly.

Disturbingly, in the context of brain injury, when patients are perceived to have contributed to their own injury, Redpath et al. found that "Increased prejudicial attitudes of qualified staff are related to a decrease in intended helping behaviour, which has the potential to impact negatively on an individual's recovery post-injury" (Redpath et al. 2010). In other words, blaming the patient for their own injury tends to decrease the intention of medical staff to help the "blameworthy" patient, with resulting negative effects on physical and psychological recovery. Physicians exhibit more prejudicial attitudes than nurses, and "have the least positive attitudes toward individuals with a head injury, regardless of the attribution of blame for the injury" (Redpath et al. 2010). Redpath and colleagues argued that the stigma experienced by survivors of brain injuries can affect recovery as well as adjustment to brain injury, and that difficulties experienced by individuals with brain injuries should be viewed less as products of deficits or impairments, and more as resulting from socially constructed factors (Redpath et al. 2010, 810).

8.5.3 Implicit Bias and Willful Ignorance

As epistemic agents, medical staff are blameworthy for failing to recognize and counteract their implicit and explicit ableist biases. Theirs is a particular type of epistemic injustice, which Gaile Pohlhaus, Jr., has called *willful hermeneutical ignorance*. Willful hermeneutical ignorance is the failure of privileged epistemic agents to acknowledge the epistemic tools and experience of the marginalized, and to remain ignorant when they could acquire knowledge that would contribute to epistemic justice.

> We need epistemic resources to make sense of our world. Because epistemic resources are maintained and developed interdependently, we need one another in order to have and use them. When epistemic agents refuse to allow the development of, or refuse to acknowledge already developed, epistemic resources for knowing the world from situations other than their own, they contribute to epistemic injustice and maintain their own ignorance about whole parts of the world. (2012)

Medical staff have unique influence, and their failure to acknowledge the perspectives and self-knowledge of disabled persons, to use epistemic resources to counteract their own biases, is an example of epistemic injustice. We could also characterize this willful hermeneutical ignorance as neglecting their epistemic duty to seek more evidence.

8.6 Withdrawal of LST as Prevention of Disability

Upstream decision-making is sometimes concerned with avoiding a prolonged but inevitable death, and sometimes concerned with *preventing* disability. It may have much in common with considerations engaged in procreative and genetic ethics about creating or preventing the existence of children with disabilities, where the choices are, again, a short life and premature death, life with disability, or no life at all. Another feature they have in common is that, frequently, certainty about specific impairments or the degree of impairment may be lacking at the point at which decisions must be made, and so the ethical risks—giving up a chance at a good, flourishing life—are similar. A feature they do not share is that in *acquired* brain injury contexts, the person in question already exists, and often has had experiences, has formed relationships, has had goals, dreams, values, desires, and beliefs, including beliefs about what counts as a good and flourishing life. That person may have much to lose whether they live or die. The individual in question in prenatal contexts is merely possible, and will experience no losses if they cease to exist or never exist at all.[10]

Sometimes individual patients with brain injuries have indicated their preferences and values about treatment and LST in case they are incapacitated by serious injury or illness. It is usually left to their families and surrogates to interpret those preferences and values in light of the circumstances, and make decisions on their behalf. Those decisions may be based on a number of considerations that include the prognosis for recovery or death, what they think the patient would want them to do (consistent with the patient's values and preferences), what is in the patient's best interests, the potential for pain and suffering, the practical and emotional effects on caregivers, and the financial and other resources available to the family or patient should they require continuing (or frequent) hospitalization, rehabilitation, and nursing care. Within that

---

[10] I assume that even embryos and fetuses, whether we consider them persons or not (see chapter 7), do not experience their lives in the way that persons who have already been born do, and do not experience any losses should their existence be cut off in the prenatal period. There is an extensive, rich, and varied bioethical literature on prenatal selection, procreative ethics, and disability, and I won't attempt to summarize it here (see, for example, Stramondo 2017; Parens and Asch 2000).

complex matrix of considerations are also the spiritual and cultural beliefs that inform and shape their lives and their decisions. Some families would never countenance withdrawing LST under any circumstances, including when the patient is diagnosed as dead by neurological criteria.

Family members are generally the default surrogate decision-makers when patients have not themselves appointed someone as a healthcare proxy. There are good reasons for this. Families have generally known the patient their entire lives, and are in the best position to know and understand the patient's values, their views about what constitutes a good and flourishing life, and their views on matters of life and death. There are, of course, exceptions. Some people have reasons for not wanting their spouses or families to make their medical decisions. Some are estranged from their families, or have values and beliefs that are not shared by their families. Some parents are, or were in the past, abusive toward their children, and may not have their best interests at heart. These are important exceptions, but family members can *usually* be relied upon to want what is best for their children, their siblings, their parents, and their spouses. They are also usually in the best position to understand the social, cultural, spiritual, material, financial, and support contexts in which patients do and will live, and how those will affect the patient's well-being in the future, as well as the impact their illness or injury might have on all of these domains. Finally, family members may themselves have a stake in the decisions they make, for they may well be the primary caregivers for the patient in the short or long term, or have financial responsibility for the patient (Johnson and Cerminara 2020). For these reasons, families have prima facie authority to make decisions on behalf of their kin, and are usually and rightly the default decision makers. (Joseph Stramondo [2017] has argued in the same vein for the prima facie decisional authority of parents making prenatal decisions.)

These considerations are mirrored in procreative contexts where parents face choices based on a prenatal diagnosis or prognosis. In the reproductive context, as in the context of patients facing an uncertain future and prognosis following a brain injury, the decisions involve whether or not an individual continues to live. For my purposes, it doesn't matter whether or not we view prenatal beings as persons. What prenatal and post-injury decisions have in common is that both can involve decisions to withdraw the means of sustaining life, whether that is life in another's body, or life in an intensive care bed. In both cases, one of the possible choices that parents or family surrogates have is termination—abortion in the prenatal context, and withdrawal of LST in the injury context. Needless to say, parents also sometimes must make the latter choice for premature or very sick neonates, or for infants and older children, including adult children.[11] And the outcome of that choice will be that the individual in question no longer exists.

The future nonexistence of the individual is what makes these choices unusual, and unusually vexing. It is difficult, at best, to square nonexistence with the interests or best interests of a person (or future person). Disability scholars have frequently criticized terminations of otherwise wanted pregnancies based on prenatal diagnosis of disability. Erik Parens and Adrienne Asch, for example, argued that these terminations are influenced by bias, a lack of information, and synecdoche, or a tendency to substitute a single characteristic of a possible person for the whole person (Parens and Asch 2000). A common critique of prenatal diagnosis and termination is that the parents making those decisions are rarely presented with adequate information—beyond a medicalized diagnosis and prognosis—to enable them to make an informed choice. This critique is also levelled at the medical model of disability, in which disability is presented only in terms of tragedy and loss. And here

---

[11] The choice to terminate is more common in the prenatal context than in the brain injury context. For example, an estimated 61 to 93 percent of pregnancies with a prenatal diagnosis of Trisomy 21 are terminated (Natoli et al. 2012).

again, the framing of such discussions may reflect implicit biases on the part of both medical staff and surrogates.[12]

> Social stigmas perpetuating myths about life with a disability being unavoidably tragic warp most people's judgment about whether a given disability will allow for an acceptable range of opportunity in any context. There is evidence that such stigmas cause non-disabled people to consistently evaluate life with disability as much more dismal than how that life is actually experienced by a disabled person. (Stramondo 2017, 484)

Stramondo was referring to procreative decisions, but he could just as easily have been referring to treatment decisions for persons with acquired or anticipated disabilities. Making either decision based on assumptions and judgments about life with disability, rather than on information about the actual lived experiences of relevantly similar disabled persons potentially depends too much on unreflective bias for decisions that are momentous, shape families and societies, and influence who exists and who does not. Such decisions should be better informed, to allow them to be more thoughtful and careful. And likewise for decisions to terminate LST in persons who already exist.

But as Stramondo noted, from the fact that many disabled persons live good and fulfilling lives, "it does not follow that every disability allows for a life in which a person can access a sufficiently broad range of life opportunities in any context" (Stramondo 2017, 484). Stramondo has described a useful and fruitful strategy for considering which kinds of parental choices are morally suspect, and which are in the range of morally permissible parental decisions about what kinds of children they create.

---

[12] In a study by Gould et al., 90 percent of genetic counselors—including those who provide prenatal counseling to parents and would-be parents—demonstrated implicit ableism as scored in the Disability Attitudes Implicit Association Test (Gould et al. 2019).

We might determine when a future disabled child is likely to have an acceptable range of life opportunities by making a judgment about whether the potential parents and surrounding community will be able to provide the accommodations the child will need to access such opportunities. This is a multidimensional question that will depend on features of the future child's physiology, but, just as importantly, the material, epistemic, and emotional resources of her parents and community. (2017, 486)

Stramondo importantly includes within the context of procreative decisions the contextual features that are unique to individuals and families. In chapter 6, I describe many of the same considerations, which can be applied to decision-making by surrogates of patients with brain injuries as they contemplate possible futures. The *All Things Considered* model of surrogate decision-making for DoC patients is one that is importantly attentive to, and permits, considerations of the unique familial, social, cultural, spiritual, financial, and individual needs and values that are present for a particular patient with a particular injury and outcome (Johnson and Cerminara 2020).

Even if we agree (and we should) with disability critiques of the medical model of disability, and agree (as we should) that much that is disabling about impairments is situated not in the individual, but in the non-ideal, unjust socio-cultural-economic contexts in which they live, it is still the case that surrogates have no option but to make decisions in those non-ideal contexts. They and the patients they decide for must be able to live with the outcomes of those decisions, in sometimes downright hostile social communities and financial circumstances. The lack of access to neurorehabilitation, or to high-quality skilled nursing facilities, or to home health aides is beyond the control of many families, but so are the sociopolitical remedies. Moreover, unlike some other disabilities, many impairments of DoC patients are simply not remediable through accommodation. It is certainly true that these patients can be kept alive and provided with medical treatment and prevention. For those who are mini-mally conscious, accommodations that facilitate social and emo-tional inclusion can be important, although, as we saw with M, the benefits may be ambiguous. DoCs are importantly different from many other disabilities. Some DoCs may specifically be incompat-ible with a range of reasonable *individual* conceptions of a good, fulfilling, and flourishing life, and so we should exercise caution in treating DoCs like paradigmatic disabilities and applying disability critiques to decisions made for patients like Terri Schiavo.

Finally, adult patients with acquired, incapacitating brain injuries and DoCs may be importantly different from some other disabled persons (and prenatal/preconception life) in another re-spect. They may have had developed and durable preferences about how they wanted their lives to go, and a conception of a good and flourishing life for themselves. Whether or not their preferences were informed by prejudicial attitudes or misconceptions about disability, or warped by myths about disability, or shaped by social, cultural, spiritual, financial, or familial factors, the same reasons for granting other individuals (including other disabled persons) autonomy and epistemic authority in making decisions about con-tinuing medical treatment, refusals of treatment, and terminations of treatment for themselves obtain. Medical decision-making by patients and surrogates is never free of all bias and motive—that is simply not a reasonable or practical standard, especially when decisions concern emotionally fraught life and death matters. We don't generally expect patients to be free of motives and sub-jectivity, and have fully informed and objective reasons for their decisions. There are not compelling reasons to think the standard should be higher for decision-making that concerns the possibility of life with a disability or a DoC. Patient preferences can properly guide surrogate decisions, and undergird surrogate decisional au-thority. Family members are usually best situated to know those preferences and to have shared circumstances and values. By some measures, the decisions will always be flawed. They may well be the best possible under the circumstances. The duties of surrogates as epistemic and moral agents must be viewed in the context of uncertainty, and their inability to do better than the best they can do.

8.6.1 All Things Considered, Again

Decisions concerning continuation or termination of LST following brain injuries must be made by surrogates who care about the lives they are deciding about, and who have an important stake in the outcome of their decisions. Their decisions will affect whether someone exists in the future with impairments and disabilities the effects of which are often difficult to predict. It is reasonable and permissible for surrogates to take an all things considered approach to those decisions, considering the social, cultural, spiritual, financial, emotional, and familial contexts in which they and the patient live, and the values and preferences the patient had. Where the epistemic duties of privileged epistemic agents like physicians and medical staff have been properly discharged, those surrogates will know and understand the uncertainty that surrounds diagnosis and prognosis, and take that into consideration alongside all other things. Their decisions will be made against the backdrop of existing just and unjust sociopolitical circumstances that are beyond the control of patients and their surrogates. Those circumstances include the availability and accessibility of rehabilitation and accommodations, which can affect the patient's life opportunities, and their prospects for well-being, and for living a good and flourishing life, a conception of which they would endorse. In other words, in making upstream decisions, surrogates cannot ignore downstream considerations, because if the patient lives, they will encounter those downstream circumstances. Nonetheless, epistemically responsible and ethically reflective decisions require careful consideration and balancing of foreseeable but uncertain upstream and downstream risks. Where patients cannot engage in that reflection themselves, there is an epistemic and ethical responsibility on the part of surrogates and their advisors—including medical staff—to honestly assess their own ableist biases, exercise epistemic humility, and decide as best they can.

8.7 Upstream/Downstream Revisited: Reinverting the Risks

The considerations in this chapter and chapter 5 suggest that the upstream/downstream risks that influence decisions to withdraw LST in neurointensive care are inverted in a worrisome way. That the risks are inverted does not mean that the decisions that are ultimately made are always wrong. It does mean that a reorienting of the risks may be needed to ensure that the decisions made are as good as they can be, all things considered.

The risks of downstream disability, and especially severe disability, are uncertain following a brain injury, but they loom large. In the hours after a brain injury, prognostication concerning future survival, recovery of consciousness, and recovery with or without impairment or deficits is underdetermined by the available empirical evidence, and thus can be overly influenced by biases, including ableism. Self-fulfilling prophecies of death add to the epistemic challenges of prognosticating. The upstream and downstream risks are certainly inverted. This is a Problem of Inductive Risk: given prognostic uncertainty, what is the appropriate epistemic standard of evidence for accepting an ethically risky prediction? The First Principle of Inductive Risk tells us that the tolerable level of epistemic risk or uncertainty should be limited by the ethical risks of being wrong. The risks of being wrong—the brain-injured patient dies and misses an opportunity to live a good and flourishing life—are quite significant, and so we ought to demand a high degree of epistemic certainty in prognosticating. That certainty may well be elusive, which is why the Second Principle of

Inductive Risk is more important to decisions about continuing and withdrawing LST in the aftermath brain injury. That principle tells us that the acceptable level of *ethical* risk should be constrained by the level of epistemic (diagnostic and prognostic) uncertainty. Again, given that the patient will certainly die and could miss out on a good and flourishing life, the ethical risks of withdrawing LST are quite significant. Accepting those risks should ideally be done only in case we have a level of epistemic certainty that is commensurate with the significance of the decision. But it is frequently the case that early prognosis cannot provide that degree of certainty, and waiting for more certainty may subject the patient to other downstream risks that they would rather have avoided if they could.

If there is a need to reinvert the risks to set things right, what might that involve? One modest and feasible possibility is that surrogate decision makers be informed of, and understand, the uncertainties and risks involved. This information would then be included in the diverse set of considerations that inform the decisions they make, to be given weight in an all things considered process. It is, I have argued, the epistemic duty of physicians and other medical staff to inform surrogates so that their decisions can consider that uncertainty and its risks.

One possible outcome of giving more weight to the fact of uncertainty is that decisions to wait and see, and to give patients more time to recover, will be more frequent. Waiting—ignoring the time pressure of the window of opportunity—can sometimes enable diagnosis and prognosis to achieve somewhat higher levels of certainty in circumstances where the patient survives. But waiting carries the downstream risk that the patient will survive in a condition they would not find acceptable. Should that happen, more, and potentially more difficult, downstream decisions about the continuation of LST will be faced by surrogates. Those include decisions, perhaps years later, to withdraw ANH. That is what happened in Terri Schiavo's case.

Given the frequency of misdiagnosis of DoCs, there remains considerable epistemic uncertainty, and so a low level of ethical risk-taking is epistemically and ethically optimal. According to the Second Principle, then, there will be circumstances in which decisions to withdraw LST—in acute brain injury, and in persistent or chronic DoCs—could be judged intolerably risky. The challenge for surrogates—one they are uniquely well suited to undertake—is to weigh the various risks and uncertainties alongside other considerations, including the wishes and values of the patient, and to decide accordingly.

8.8 Holding the Tension

I mean Negative Capability, *that is when man is capable of being in uncertainties, Mysteries, doubts, without any irritable reaching after fact & reason . . .*

—John Keats, in an 1818 letter to his brothers[13]

Additional information and/or time may or may not influence surrogate decisions to the degree epistemic demands would warrant. It may not change their decisions in the ways those who worry about the undue influence of myths and misinformation about disability would prefer. In M's case, her family sought treatment and rehabilitative therapy for several years before concluding that M's life was not one she would find acceptable or want to live. So, too, did Terri Schiavo's husband. The extent to which these decisions are deeply personal, significant, emotional, and fraught should not be underestimated, nor should surrogates facing these singularly

---

[13] Keats attributed this negative capability to William Shakespeare. (Shakespeare's son Hamnet died at the age of 11, at roughly the same time that his father achieved success as a playwright.)

terrible choices have their feet held to the fire to ensure epistemically or ethically consistent and unassailable decisions.

Implicit in the label *vegetative state* is the idea that unconscious
individuals are less than human, or no longer persons. Such views
about the VS/UWS are commonly endorsed by medical staff,
judges, bioethicists, and the public, including family members of
patients. Forcefully rejecting the implication that disabled persons
are *less than*, whether that means less than non-disabled persons, or
less than human, has been an important achievement of disability
scholarship and activism. Persons in the VS/UWS, however, do not
fit easily in even a capacious understanding of disability. While it
is easy to imagine and easy to find examples of disabled persons
living good and flourishing lives, it is difficult to imagine that being
chronically unaware aligns with many individuals' conceptions
of a good and flourishing life. The diverse goods of life, small and
large, cannot be enjoyed or appreciated absent awareness. That is
very different, however, from saying that unconscious individuals
are no longer persons, or are persons of a lesser status. What we owe
to profoundly impaired persons like those with DoCs is what we
owe to others: care, careful consideration of their preferences and
interests, and respect for their personhood. It is only by deciding
and acting in accordance with those moral duties that we can hope
to do what is right and best.

9

Responding to Uncertainty

Beyond Disorders of Consciousness

Patients with disorders of consciousness (DoCs) have an impaired ability to communicate. This makes it exceedingly difficult to assess their needs and wants. Even when they retain some capacity to speak or gesture, their behaviors and verbalizations can be ambiguous. M occasionally uttered intelligible words—*what* and *bloody hell*—and she sometimes appeared to cry, but her intentions and the meaning of her utterances were very much open to interpretation. We can easily summon other vulnerable persons in similar situations, including infants and persons with advanced Alzheimer's dementia. Some of the same uncertainties that vex decision-making for DoC patients make it difficult for those others as well. And we can ask some of the same questions. What would this person want us to do, if they could tell us? What is in their best interest? Are they suffering? What does the future hold for them? *What should we do?*

In previous chapters I discuss a few other medical contexts, beyond brain injuries and DoCs, where the principles of inductive risk can be useful in taking the measure of, and attenuating, epistemic and ethical uncertainty. One is prenatal testing, where the risks and considerations are sometimes similar to those found in the context of DoCs. There, the First Principle of Inductive Risk argues for a low level of epistemic uncertainty given the risks. The other case involves the use of the power morcellator, a surgical tool, to remove uterine fibroids. There the epistemic uncertainties are straightforward—it cannot be known prior to removal if a fibroid is benign or contains hidden malignancy. Both the high level of uncertainty and the severity of the risk argue against the use of power morcellators when the principles of inductive risk are applied. Considerations of epistemic distributive justice in both cases also place demands on medical staff as epistemic agents.

I turn now to a few other contexts where there is intersecting, interacting epistemic and ethical uncertainty. My aim is to highlight some quite different scenarios in which the ethics of uncertainty might be helpful. This is in no way intended to be an exhaustive treatment of the applicability of the ethics of uncertainty. There are numerous contexts where there is a need for decisive action in the presence of unavoidable epistemic uncertainty. The First and Second Principles of Inductive Risk provide us with rough guides for managing the uncertainty in the presence of risk, and risk in the presence of uncertainty. Another important element of the ethics of uncertainty is the focus on epistemic duties, including duties to seek knowledge where there is uncertainty, and to promote epistemic *distributive* justice. The last piece is recognizing the necessity and permissibility of considering an expansive array of entangled personal, interpersonal, and familial values, social and cultural facts and values, resource needs, and epistemic uncertainties—many of which may be in tension—in making ethically risky decisions. All of these enter the arena in decisions involving DoC patients. Some will be more important than others in different contexts.

9.1 Pain

Pain, like consciousness, is a first-person accessible, subjectively phenomenal experience, the quality and quantity of which are hard to put into words. It isn't objectively measurable or visible, although the cause of pain might be.[1] A broken bone, a purple bruise, and an angry rash all can be painful, and the cause visible but not the

---

[1] Tor Wager and colleagues reported that they had found a neurologic signature of pain using functional magnetic resonance (fMRI). They identified a pattern of fMRI

pain associated with it. Not every pain reveals itself objectively. As Buchman, Ho, and Goldberg observed, pain can be epistemically inaccessible in a way that defies medical epistemic "frameworks of clinical correlation and pathological anatomy":

> Especially in chronic pain discourse, the natural object does not always reveal the truth of the assertion: the patient's symptoms do not correlate with any visible scientific object. Thus, pain defies the process of clinical correlation that is central to the anatomo-clinical method. . . . Many, if not most, kinds of chronic pain cannot be correlated with any underlying pathology. (2017)

As a consequence, when reported pain has no identified, objective, physical correlate, a pain sufferer may not be trusted, either as a competent reporter or as a truthful one. A physician may be suspicious of the patient's motives—they may think the patient is malingering, or drug-seeking. Persons from socially marginalized groups are more likely to encounter this kind of prejudicial stereotyping, in addition to the many other health-related and healthcare disparities they experience (Green et al. 2003).

It was shockingly recently that infant pain was experimentally "proven" to exist. Kanwaljeet Anand, a neonatologist in the United Kingdom, observed that preterm neonates frequently returned from major surgeries exhibiting symptoms of shock, and it required hours of medical intervention to stabilize them. Once he learned that they were not receiving anesthesia during surgery, he attributed their physiological condition to the immense pain they experienced, and set about proving it experimentally (Anand, Sippell, and Green 1987). Anesthetizing neonates is challenging and risky, and the medical consensus that they could not feel pain because their nervous systems were underdeveloped made it possible

activity across brain regions associated with heat-induced pain in healthy subjects. They also were able to discriminate fairly well between physical pains and social pains—the subjects had all recently experienced a painful romantic breakup and rejection, and they were shown pictures of their ex-partners to elicit "social pain" (Wager et al. 2013).

to perform surgeries without the added risks of anesthesia. Anand and colleagues showed that there are other significant risks associated with the severe procedural pain experienced by neonates. To this day, however, neonatal pain remains undertreated.

And recall Kate Bainbridge's reports of the pain she experienced, and her unheeded screams.

Pain sufferers encounter testimonial injustice because of the subjectivity, invisibility, and objective uncertainty of pain. The antidote to testimonial injustice is epistemic humility. Epistemic humility here can include trusting the testimony of patients (in whatever form it takes), and acknowledging the limits of one's own knowledge and the inescapable epistemic uncertainty of pain. Moreover, the principles of inductive risk can help us to properly balance the epistemic and ethical risks that include overtreating and undertreating pain, both of which can cause harm and suffering.

9.2 Medical Research: Vaccine Development

The prototype for the First Principle can be found in Rudner's discussion of inductive risk in science. It should be no surprise that there are a range of scientific contexts in which the principles of inductive risk can be utilized. Inductive risk exists because any scientific hypothesis can turn out to be wrong, and no instance or accumulation of evidence can establish the correctness of an hypothesis with certainty. As Rudner stated it, "Clearly how great a risk one is willing to take of being wrong in accepting or rejecting the hypothesis will depend upon how seriously in the typically ethical sense one views the consequences of making a mistake" (Rudner 1953). That is, normative judgments are needed—decisions about accepting scientific hypotheses are decisions about acceptable epistemic standards, but those epistemic standards are not free-floating and unencumbered by considerations of the effects of being wrong. We can't make those epistemic choices in an ethical vacuum, where the ethically relevant impacts of our decisions are excluded from consideration. If our epistemic choices carry the risk of harms or deaths, then that must influence our decisions about the level of uncertainty that is acceptable. Scientists don't make epistemic choices without also making ethical choices, by intention or by default.

When the first COVID-19 vaccines were initially approved for emergency use at the end of 2020, as a global pandemic raged, the decisions by regulatory agencies considered evidence of safety and efficacy—both of which are to some extent uncertain and individually variable. But the risks of not accepting the evidence (and the vaccines), also included quite certain, well-documented risks of the pandemic: infection, illness, disability, and deaths, as well as negative societal effects. The weight given to the inductive inferences that the vaccines were safe and effective can be measured against the weight of the ethically significant risks of both acceptance and non-acceptance. The epistemic and ethical risks form a thorny thicket when there are multidimensional considerations that include the risks of accepting and *not accepting* inferences and the hypotheses they support. It's not simply calculating utilities, or, as in the balance sheet model used in M's case, totting up the *fors* and *againsts*. Such scenarios, with multiple considerations weighing for and against accepting epistemic standards, are more common than not, including in science.[2]

---

[2] It should surprise no one that many decisions in science involve value judgments. The very choices about what scientific goals to pursue, what things to study, what problems to tackle, what scientific research to fund, what methods to use (e.g., whether and how nonhuman animals and human subjects will be used), and how scientific innovation and discovery will be used—involve matters of value. Even the decision to pursue research to satisfy one's own curiosity places value on the satisfaction of curiosity. As Douglas argued, "value-free science is inadequate science," and non-epistemic values should also inform "the internal stages of science: choice of methodology, characterization of data, and interpretation of result" (Douglas 2000, 559).

During the COVID-19 pandemic, decisions to accelerate the pace of vaccine research, to divert scientific resources from other research programs, to grant Emergency Use Authorization to vaccines, all involved value judgments that weighed the benefits against the risks.

What does that mean for applying the principles of inductive risk?
It means it's always complicated.

9.3 Nonhuman Animals

At several points in the book I mention nonhuman animals. At
present, nonhuman animals are exploited and killed for numerous
reasons by humans: they are killed in the billions annually for food
(or the trillions, when fish are counted); they are killed for their
fur, feathers, and skins; they are killed because they pose threats
to other animals used for food (e.g., wolves who prey on livestock,
bison who can spread brucellosis to cattle, and through cattle to
humans); they are killed for sport. Many more are killed by human
practices like deforestation that cause habitat loss. Countless
millions (mostly mice, but many other species as well) are used
and killed for medical and industrial experimentation and testing.
Others are held captive in zoos, aquaria, theme parks, and shopping
malls for human entertainment. As Rachels recounted, when the
idea of moral status was introduced in the 1970s, the treatment of
animals was one of several issues that philosophers thought might
be resolved once we got moral status sorted out.

I don't think we'll get moral status sorted out, and if we did,
I don't think it would help. Can the ethics of uncertainty help?

There are many and various epistemic uncertainties concerning
nonhuman animals. Consciousness is not one of them. There is
very considerable evidence that very many species of nonhuman
animals are sentient and conscious. They feel pain, they engage in
complex, purposeful, intentional behaviors, they plan, they think,
they have emotions. Some are moral agents. There are some edge
cases where there is less certainty, and where there is a reasonable possibility that the animals in question—for example corals,
sponges, oysters—might not be conscious. Not in the way that
creatures like mammals are conscious, to be sure. There is some

question about insect consciousness, although the complexity and intentionality of some insect behaviors suggests that they could be. An interesting hypothesis about insects is that they are conscious, but not sentient—they don't appear to experience pain. (Pain is only one type of suffering, however. Perhaps insects can be anxious? Fearful? Angry?) Godfrey-Smith would say that animal subjectivity is everywhere—animals are *selves*. There is something it is like to be them (Godfrey-Smith 2020).

Earlier I rejected the Consciousness Criterion and consciousness as a necessary condition of personhood or mattering morally. It's not that consciousness doesn't matter at all—it surely does matter as a feature of how our lives go, and whether they go well or ill. One thing consciousness makes possible is suffering. Conscious creatures can suffer, they can experience pain, sorrow, and frustration, and they can experience joy, satisfaction, and pleasure.

In biomedical research involving animals, the standard justification for using animals in ways that cause them to suffer is the benefit to humans. For thousands of years, animals have been used as substitutes where using humans was prohibited by taboos or, more recently, by regulation. Animal models are typically used in early stages of research and discovery, to test out hypotheses, to test toxicity of new drugs, to test the safety of devices, and to test efficacy. But nonhuman animals are not humans, so research must eventually proceed to human subjects once the thing being investigated is deemed likely to be safe and likely to be effective. Even after several species have been used to study, say, a drug, it is still possible for that drug to prove unsafe or ineffective in humans. This problem is well documented and known to the scientific community. The so-called attrition rate—the rate of drugs that fail to translate from animals to humans—is over 90 percent (Pound and Ritskes-Hoitinga 2018). As one example, despite thousands of experiments, with multiple species, to date only a single therapeutic drug for strokes has been developed (Johnson 2020b). That drug, tPA, was developed using a rabbit model and was approved in 1996.

Since then, nothing. There have been more than a hundred human clinical trials of dozens of drugs, none of which has succeeded.

There are many stages in the lengthy process of developing hypotheses, designing experiments, and reviewing and approving research proposals where inductive risks are present. I focus here on just one. In the United States and other countries, research using animals must be approved by an ethical review board (known as Institutional Animal Care and Use Committees, or IACUCs, in the United States). IACUCs judge whether the animals used, and the methods and protocols employed, are in keeping with animal welfare regulations that require minimizing pain and distress to the extent possible while meeting the needs of the experiment (Pound and Nicol 2018). That this is done is already an admission that animals are sentient, that animals matter morally (at least to some extent), and that animal welfare and animal suffering matter and should be minimized. That much is baked in, and we need not question it. One thing IACUCs are not asked to do is judge whether the supposed benefits of the research outweigh the potential harms to animals. That is a matter of inductive risk. There are known risks of harm (including induced illness, pain, and death) to the animals. Those are ethical risks, if animals are moral patients who matter morally, and that they are is also acknowledged by animal welfare regulations. The benefits of animal research are epistemically uncertain, just as any untested hypothesis is uncertain. Experience suggests that about 90 percent of investigations with animals can be expected to fail either before or when human studies occur, but it can be higher (as in stroke research), or lower, depending on the specific research. (Those failures pose risks to humans as well—including risks of toxicity and serious adverse events from drugs that appeared safe in animals.)

Suppose an IACUC considered inductive risk and applied the principles of inductive risk to decisions about which experiments were permissible. Given known ethical risks of suffering and death for the animals used, and given epistemically uncertain benefits (for example, less than 1 in 1,000 of the stroke treatments tested in animals have worked in humans), this seems a clear case where the First Principle of Inductive Risk would often indicate an unacceptable level of epistemic risk measured against the ethical risks. If the ethical risks constrain the level of acceptable epistemic risks, such experiments should not proceed. A possible remedy is to reduce the epistemic risks (without creating more ethical risks). Applying the Second Principle, similarly, indicates that the ethical risks are *too risky* to undertake given the level of epistemic uncertainty. Again, experiments where this is the case should not proceed.

This does not necessarily mean that all research with animals is ruled out—it is in principle possible to achieve the right balance of risks by modifying either the epistemic or ethical risks—but it rules out a great deal of research using animals. Consideration of inductive risks is not currently in the ethical or scientific toolboxes used in the review and approval of research with animals. It should be. The ethical and epistemic risks are entangled and intersecting, and by evaluating inductive risk, both scientists and ethical review bodies can make decisions that are better informed by the relevant risks and uncertainties, and that are consistent with both their epistemic and moral duties.

9.4 Untangling

The scenarios in which there is epistemic uncertainty and ethical risks are many and varied. Implementing the ethics of uncertainty will emphasize different aspects of the overall scheme as is needed in specific cases and contexts.

Where complexity prevails, our impulse is to simplify, cut through the thicket rather than untangle it. Seeking simplicity or heuristics to aid decision-making are not strategies that can be expected to make decisions or decision-making *better*. They make decisions simpler for the sake of simplicity, and perhaps quicker.

Applying the First and Second Principles of Inductive Risk, attending to epistemic justice, and considering *all things* do not make decisions simpler or quicker, and I see no reason to think they will always make them easier. So why bother?

We should bother because in situations where there are ethically important risks that fall out of errors, such as harms and deaths, as there are in medicine, we should avoid those risks when we can. In so doing, we can aspire to fulfill our obligations as epistemic and moral agents. As we should.

Bibliography

Academy of Medical Royal Colleges. "A Code of Practice for the Diagnosis and Confirmation of Death" (London: Academy of Medical Royal Colleges, 2008). https://www.aomrc.org.uk/reports-guidance/ukdec-reports-and-guidance/code-practice-diagnosis-confirmation-death/.

ADA Watch, ADAPT, AIMMM—Advancing Independence, Center for Self Determination, Center on Human Policy, Citizens United Resisting Euthanasia (CURE), Disability Rights Center, Disability Rights Education & Defense Fund, Disability Rights Project of the Public Interest Law Center of Philadelphia, Hospice Patients Alliance, National Catholic Partnership on Disability, National Coalition for Disability Rights, National Coalition on Self-Determination, National Council on Independent Living, National Disabled Students Union, National Down Syndrome Congress, National Organization on Disability, National Spinal Cord Injury Association, Not Dead Yet, Self Advocates Becoming Empowered (SABE), TASH, World Association of Persons with disAbilities, and World Institute on Disability. "Issues Surrounding Terri Schindler-Schiavo Are Disability Rights Issues, Say National Disability Organizations." *Ragged Edge Magazine,* 2003. http://www.raggededgemagazine.com/schiavostatement.html.

Albrecht, Gary L., Katherine D. Seelman, and Michael Bury. *Handbook of Disability Studies.* Thousand Oaks, CA: SAGE Publications, 2001.

Alpers, Lise-Merete. "Distrust and Patients in Intercultural Healthcare: A Qualitative Interview Study." *Nursing Ethics* 25, no. 3 (2018): 313–323.

Alston, William P. "The Deontological Conception of Epistemic Justification." *Philosophical Perspectives* 2 (1988): 257–299.

Anand, Kanwaljeet J. S., W. G. Sippell, and A. Aynsley Green. "Randomised Trial of Fentanyl Anaesthesia in Preterm Babies Undergoing Surgery: Effects on the Stress Response." *The Lancet* 329, no. 8527 (1987): 243–248.

Andrews, Keith, Lesley Murphy, Ros Munday, and Clare Littlewood. "Misdiagnosis of the Vegetative State: Retrospective Study in a Rehabilitation Unit." *BMJ: British Medical Journal* 313, no. 7048 (1996): 13–16.

Andrews, Kristin, Gary Comstock, G. K. D. Crozier, Sue Donaldson, Andrew Fenton, Tyler John, L. Syd M Johnson, Robert Jones, Will Kymlicka, and Letitia Meynell. *Chimpanzee Rights: The Philosophers' Brief.* New York: Routledge, 2019.

Anke, Audny, Nada Andelic, Toril Skandsen, Rein Knoph, Tiina Ader, Unn Manskow, Solrun Sigurdardottir, and Cecilie Røe. "Functional Recovery and Life Satisfaction in the First Year after Severe Traumatic Brain Injury: A Prospective Multicenter Study of a Norwegian National Cohort." *The Journal of Head Trauma Rehabilitation* 30, no. 4 (2015): E38–E49.

Appel, Jacob M. "Rational Rationing vs. Irrational Rationing: The Struggle for the Legacy of Ruben Betancourt." *HuffPost,* June 23, 2010, https://www.huffpost.com/entry/rational-rationing-vs-irr_b_622057.

Appelbaum, Paul S., and Thomas G. Gutheil. " 'Rotting with Their Rights on': Constitutional Theory and Clinical Reality in Drug Refusal by Psychiatric Patients." *Bulletin of the American Academy of Psychiatry and the Law* 7, no. 3 (1979): 306–315.

Aristotle. *The Basic Works of Aristotle.* New York: Random House, 1941.

Asai, Atsushi, Munetaka Maekawa, Ichiro Akiguchi, Tsuguya Fukui, Yasuhiko Miura, Noboru Tanabe, and Shunichi Fukuhara. "Survey of Japanese Physicians' Attitudes Towards the Care of Adult Patients in Persistent Vegetative State." *Journal of Medical Ethics* 25, no. 4 (1999): 302–308.

Asch, Adrienne. "Disability, Bioethics and Human Rights." In *Handbook of Disability Studies,* edited by Gary L. Albrecht, Katherine D. Seelman, and Michael Bury, 297-326. Thousand Oaks, CA: SAGE Publications, 2001.

Asch, Adrienne. "Recognizing Death While Affirming Life: Can End of Life Reform Uphold a Disabled Person's Interest in Continued Life?" *The Hastings Center Report* 35, no.6 (2005): S31–S36.

Bailey, Moya, and Izetta Autumn Mobley. "Work in the Intersections: A Black Feminist Disability Framework." *Gender & Society* 33, no. 1 (2019): 19–40.

Barnato, Amber E., and Robert M. Arnold. "The Effect of Emotion and Physician Communication Behaviors on Surrogates' Life-Sustaining Treatment Decisions: A Randomized Simulation Experiment." *Critical Care Medicine* 41, no. 7 (2013): 1686–1691.

Barnes, Elizabeth. *The Minority Body: A Theory of Disability.* New York: Oxford University Press, 2016.

Batavia, Andrew I. "Disability and Physician-Assisted Suicide." *New England Journal of Medicine* 336 (1997): 1671–1673.

Batavia, Andrew I. "The New Paternalism: Portraying People with Disabilities as an Oppressed Minority." *Journal of Disability Policy Studies* 12, no. 2 (2001): 107–113.

Batavia, Andrew I. "Disability Rights in the Third Stage of the Independent Living Movement: Disability Community Consensus, Dissention, and the Future of Disability Policy." *Stanford Law & Policy Review* 14 (2003): 347.

Bayne, Tim, Jakob Hohwy, and Adrian M. Owen. "Are There Levels of Consciousness?" *Trends in Cognitive Sciences* 20, no. 6 (2016): 405–413.

Bayne, Tim, Jakob Hohwy, and Adrian M. Owen. "Reforming the Taxonomy in Disorders of Consciousness." *Annals of Neurology* 82, no. 6 (2017): 866–872.

Beecher, Henry, Raymond Adams, Clifford Barger, William Curran, Derek Denny-Brown, Dana Farnsworth, Jordi Folch-Pi, Everett Mendelsohn, John

Merrill, Joseph Murray, Ralph Potter, Robert Schwab, and William Sweet. "A Definition of Irreversible Coma: Report of the Ad Hoc Committee of the Harvard Medical School to Examine the Definition of Brain Death." *JAMA* 205, no. 6 (1968): 337–340.

Bekinschtein, T., J. Niklison, L. Sigman, F.R.L.J.A. Manes, R. Leiguarda, J. Armony, A. Owen, S. Carpintiero, and L. Olmos. "Emotion Processing in the Minimally Conscious State." *Journal of Neurology, Neurosurgery & Psychiatry* 75, no. 5 (2004): 788–788.

Belmont Commission. *The Belmont Report: Ethical Principles and Guidelines for the Protection of Human Subjects of Research*. Washington, DC: Belmont Commission, 1978.

Bentham, Jeremy. *An Introduction to the Principles of Morals and Legislation*. Oxford, UK: Clarendon Press, 1907.

Bernat, James L. "A Defense of the Whole-Brain Concept of Death." *The Hastings Center Report* 28, no. 2 (1998): 14–23.

Bernat, James L. "The Biophilosophical Basis of Whole-Brain Death." *Social Philosophy & Policy* 19, no. 2 (2002a): 324.

Bernat, James L. "Questions Remaining about the Minimally Conscious State." *Neurology* 58, no. 3 (2002b): 337–338.

Bito, Seiji, and Atsushi Asai. "Attitudes and Behaviors of Japanese Physicians Concerning Withholding and Withdrawal of Life-Sustaining Treatment for End-of-life Patients: Results from an Internet Survey." *BMC Medical Ethics* 8, no. 7 (2007).

Block, Ned. "On a Confusion About a Function of Consciousness." *Behavioral and Brain Sciences* 18, no. 2 (1995): 227–247.

Block, Ned. " Concepts of Consciousness." In *Philosophy of Mind: Classical and Contemporary Readings,* edited by David J. Chalmers, 206–218. Oxford, UK: Oxford University Press, 2002.

Blouin v. Spitzer, 213 F. Supp. 2d 184 (N.D.N.Y. 2002).

Blumenfeld, Hal. "Consciousness and Epilepsy: Why Are Patients with Absence Seizures Absent?" *Progress in Brain Research* 150 (2005): 271–286.

Boly, Mélanie, Marie-Elisabeth Faymonville, Caroline Schnakers, Philippe Peigneux, Bernard Lambermont, Christophe Phillips, Patrizio Lancellotti, Andre Luxen, Maurice Lamy, and Gustave Moonen. "Perception of Pain in the Minimally Conscious State with PET Activation: An Observational Study." *The Lancet Neurology* 7, no. 11 (2008): 1013–1020.

Bor, Daniel. "Advances in the Scientific Investigation of Consciousness." In *Brain Function and Responsiveness in Disorders of Consciousness*, edited by Martin M. Monti and Walter G. Sannita, 13–24. Cham: Springer, 2016.

Bosslet, Gabriel T., Thaddeus M. Pope, Gordon D. Rubenfeld, Bernard Lo, Robert D. Truog, Cynda H. Rushton, J. Randall Curtis, Dee W. Ford, Molly Osborne, and Cheryl Misak. "An Official ATS/AACN/ACCP/ ESICM/SCCM Policy Statement: Responding to Requests for Potentially

Inappropriate Treatments in Intensive Care Units." *American Journal of Respiratory and Critical Care Medicine* 191, no. 11 (2015): 1318–1330.

Brock, Dan W. "Justice and the Severely Demented Elderly." *The Journal of Medicine and Philosophy: A Forum for Bioethics and Philosophy of Medicine* 13, no. 1 (1988): 73–99.

Brody, Baruch. "The Morality of Abortion." In *Contemporary Issues in Bioethics,* edited by Tom Beauchamp and Leroy Walters, 240–250. Belmont, CA: Wadsworth, 1982.

Bruno, Marie-Aurélie, Jan L. Bernheim, Didier Ledoux, Frédéric Pellas, Athena Demertzi, and Steven Laureys. "A Survey on Self-Assessed Well-Being in a Cohort of Chronic Locked-in Syndrome Patients: Happy Majority, Miserable Minority." *BMJ Open* 1, no. 1 (2011): e000039.

Bruno, Marie-Aurélie, Audrey Vanhaudenhuyse, Aurore Thibaut, Gustave Moonen, and Steven Laureys. "From Unresponsive Wakefulness to Minimally Conscious PLUS and Functional Locked-in Syndromes: Recent Advances in Our Understanding of Disorders of Consciousness." *Journal of Neurology* 258, no. 7 (2011): 1373–1384.

Buchman, Daniel Z., Anita Ho, and Daniel S. Goldberg. "Investigating Trust, Expertise, and Epistemic Injustice in Chronic Pain." *Journal of Bioethical Inquiry* 14, no. 1 (2017): 31–42.

Carruthers, Peter. "The Problem of Animal Consciousness." *Proceedings and Addresses of the APA* 92 (2018): 179–205.

Cerminara, Kathy L., and Kenneth W. Goodman. "Key Events in the Case of Theresa Marie Schiavo," https://bioethics.miami.edu/clinical-and-research-ethics/terri-schiavo-project/index.html.

Cha, Ariana Eunjung. "Quadriplegic Man's Death from COVID-19 Spotlights Questions of Disability, Race and Family." *The Washington Post,* July 5, 2020, https://www.washingtonpost.com/health/2020/07/05/coronavirus-disability-death/.

Chalmers, David J. "What Is a Neural Correlate of Consciousness?" In *Neural Correlates of Consciousness: Empirical and Conceptual Questions,* edited by Thomas Metzinger, 17–40. Cambridge, MA: MIT Press, 2000.

Chiang, Harriet. "New Twist in Cases over Right to Die / Patient Is in Twilight State, Not in a Coma." *SFGate,* May 30, 2001, https://www.sfgate.com/news/article/New-twist-in-cases-over-right-to-die-Patient-is-2915721.php.

Clifford, William K. "The Ethics of Belief." Originally published in *Contemporary Review,* 1877. https://people.brandeis.edu/~teuber/Clifford_ethics.pdf

Coady, David. "Two Concepts of Epistemic Injustice." *Episteme* 7, no. 2 (2010): 101–113.

Cochrane, Thomas I. "Unnecessary Time Pressure in Refusal of Life-Sustaining Therapies: Fear of Missing the Opportunity to Die." *The American Journal of Bioethics* 9, no. 4 (2009): 47–54.

Conley, Zachary C., Truston J. Bodine, Andrew Chou, and Lynn Zechiedrich. "Wicked: The Untold Story of Ciprofloxacin." *PLOS Pathogens* 14, no. 3 (2018): e1006805.

Coppola, Kristen M., Peter H. Ditto, Joseph H. Danks, and William D. Smucker. "Accuracy of Primary Care and Hospital-Based Physicians' Predictions of Elderly Outpatients' Treatment Preferences with and without Advance Directives." *Archives of Internal Medicine* 161, no. 3 (2001): 431–440.

Côte, Nicolas, Alexis F. Turgeon, François Lauzier, Lynne Moore, Damon C. Scales, Francis Bernard, Ryan Zarychanski, Karen E. A. Burns, Maureen O. Meade, and David Zygun. "Factors Associated with the Withdrawal of Life-Sustaining Therapies in Patients with Severe Traumatic Brain Injury: A Multicenter Cohort Study." *Neurocritical Care* 18, no. 1 (2013): 154–160.

Cowey, Alan. "Current Awareness: Spotlight on Consciousness." *Developmental Medicine & Child Neurology* 39, no. 1 (1997): 54–62.

Cowey, Alan. "The Blindsight Saga." *Experimental Brain Research* 200, no. 1 (2010): 3–24.

Cowey, Alan, and Petra Stoerig. "Blindsight in Monkeys." *Nature* 373, no. 6511 (1995): 247–249.

Cribb, Robert. "Family, Doctors Battle over 'Do Not Resuscitate' Order." *The Toronto Star*, October 25, 2010, https://www.thestar.com/life/health_wellness/2010/10/25/family_doctors_battle_over_do_not_resuscitate_order.html.

Crisci, Claudio. "The Ultimate Curse." *Journal of Medical Ethics* 21, no. 5 (1995): 277–280.

Cruse, Damian, Srivas Chennu, Camille Chatelle, Tristan A. Bekinschtein, Davinia Fernández-Espejo, John D. Pickard, Steven Laureys, and Adrian M. Owen. "Bedside Detection of Awareness in the Vegetative State: A Cohort Study." *The Lancet* 378, no. 9809 (2011): 2088–2094.

Cruzan ex rel. Cruzan v. Director, Missouri Department of Health, 497 U.S. 261, 110 S. Ct. 2841 (1990).

DeGrazia, David. *Taking Animals Seriously: Mental Life and Moral Status*. New York: Cambridge University Press, 1996.

Dijkers, Marcel P. "Quality of Life after Traumatic Brain Injury: A Review of Research Approaches and Findings." *Archives of Physical Medicine and Rehabilitation* 85 (2004): 21–35.

Douglas, Heather. "Inductive Risk and Values in Science." *Philosophy of Science* 67, no. 4 (2000): 559–579.

Dovidio, John F., Lisa Pagotto, and Michelle R. Hebl. "Implicit Attitudes and Discrimination Against People with Physical Disabilities." In *Disability and Aging Discrimination: Perspectives in Law and Psychology*, edited by Richard L. Wiener and Steven L. Willborn, 157–183. New York: Springer, 2011.

Dresser, Rebecca S., and John A. Robertson. "Quality of Life and Non-Treatment Decisions for Incompetent Patients: A Critique of the Orthodox Approach." *Law, Medicine and Health Care* 17, no. 3 (1989): 234–244.

Dworkin, Ronald. *Life's Dominion: An Argument about Abortion, Euthanasia, and Individual Freedom.* New York: Vintage, 1994.

Edelman, Gerald M. "Building a Picture of the Brain." *Annals of the New York Academy of Sciences* 882, no. 1 (1999): 68–89.

Edlow, Brian L., Joseph T. Giacino, Ronald E. Hirschberg, Jason Gerrard, Ona Wu, and Leigh R. Hochberg. "Unexpected Recovery of Function after Severe Traumatic Brain Injury: The Limits of Early Neuroimaging-based Outcome Prediction." *Neurocritical Care* 19, no. 3 (2013): 364–375.

Eisenberg, Jon B., and J. Clark Kelso. "The Robert Wendland Case." *The Western Journal of Medicine* 176, no. 2 (2002): 124.

Evans, Leah R., Elizabeth A. Boyd, Grace Malvar, Latifat Apatira, John M. Luce, Bernard Lo, and Douglas B. White. "Surrogate Decision-Makers' Perspectives on Discussing Prognosis in the Face of Uncertainty." *American Journal of Respiratory and Critical Care Medicine* 179, no. 1 (2009): 48–53.

Eze, Michael. *Intellectual History in Contemporary South Africa.* Berlin: Springer, 2016.

Fagerlin, Angela, Peter H. Ditto, Joseph H. Danks, and Renate M. Houts. "Projection in Surrogate Decisions about Life-Sustaining Medical Treatments." *Health Psychology* 20, no. 3 (2001): 166–175.

Farisco, Michele, and Kathinka Evers. "The Ethical Relevance of the Unconscious." *Philosophy, Ethics, and Humanities in Medicine* 12, no. 1 (2017): 11.

Feinberg, William M., and Peggy C. Ferry. "A Fate Worse Than Death: The Persistent Vegetative State in Childhood." *American Journal of Diseases of Children* 138, no. 2 (1984): 128–130.

Feltz, Adam, and Stephanie Samayoa. "Heuristics and Life-Sustaining Treatments." *Journal of Bioethical Inquiry* 9, no. 4 (2012): 443–455.

Fergusson, Andrew. "Letter to the Editor." *British Medical Journal* 305 (1992): 1506.

Fernández-Espejo, Davinia, Tristan Bekinschtein, Martin M. Monti, John D. Pickard, Carme Junque, Martin R. Coleman, and Adrian M. Owen. "Diffusion Weighted Imaging Distinguishes the Vegetative State from the Minimally Conscious State." *Neuroimage* 54, no. 1 (2011): 103–112.

Fins, Joseph J. *Rights Come to Mind: Brain Injury, Ethics, and the Struggle for Consciousness.* New York: Cambridge University Press, 2015.

Fins, Joseph J., and Megan S. Wright. "Rights Language and Disorders of Consciousness: A Call for Advocacy." *Brain Injury* 32, no. 5 (2018): 670–674.

Fischer, David B., and Robert D. Truog. "The Problems with Fixating on Consciousness in Disorders of Consciousness." *American Journal of Bioethics Neuroscience* 8, no. 3 (2017): 135–140.

FitzGerald, Chloë, and Samia Hurst. "Implicit Bias in Healthcare Professionals: A Systematic Review." *BMC Medical Ethics* 18, no. 1 (2017): 19, https://doi.org/10.1186/s12910-017-0179-8.

Fletcher, Joseph. "Indicators of Humanhood: A Tentative Profile of Man." *The Hastings Center Report* 2, no. 5 (1972): 1–4.

Fletcher, Joseph F. "Four Indicators of Humanhood: The Enquiry Matures." *The Hastings Center Report* 4, no. 6 (1974): 4–7.

Food & Drug Administration. *Final Guidance: Product Labeling for Laparoscopic Power Morcellators*. Washington, DC: Food & Drug Administration, 2020.

Fricker, Miranda. *Epistemic Injustice: Power and the Ethics of Knowing*. Oxford, UK: Oxford University Press, 2007.

Fricker, Miranda. "Epistemic Justice as a Condition of Political Freedom?" *Synthese* 190, no. 7 (2013): 1317–1332.

Gadbois, Simon, and Catherine Reeve. "Canine Olfaction: Scent, Sign, and Situation." In *Domestic Dog Cognition and Behavior: The Scientific Study of Canis familiaris*, edited by Alexandra Horowitz, 3–29. Berlin: Springer, 2014.

Geurts, Marjolein, Malcolm R. Macleod, Ghislaine J. M. W. van Thiel, Jan van Gijn, L. Jaap Kappelle, and H. Bart van der Worp. "End-of-Life Decisions in Patients with Severe Acute Brain Injury." *The Lancet Neurology* 13, no. 5 (2014): 515–524.

Giacino, J. T., S. Ashwal, N. Childs, R. Cranford, B. Jennett, D. I. Katz, J. P. Kelly, J. H. Rosenberg, J. Whyte, R. D. Zafonte, and N. D. Zasler. "The Minimally Conscious State: Definition and Diagnostic Criteria." *Neurology* 58, no. 3 (2002): 349–353.

Giacino, J. T., M. Sherer, A. Christoforou, P. Maurer-Karattup, F. M. Hammond, D. Long, and E. Bagiella. "Behavioral Recovery and Early Decision Making in Patients with Prolonged Disturbance in Consciousness after Traumatic Brain Injury." *Journal of Neurotrauma* 37, no. 2 (2020): 357–365.

Giacino, Joseph T., Douglas I. Katz, Nicholas D. Schiff, John Whyte, Eric J. Ashman, Stephen Ashwal, Richard Barbano, Flora M. Hammond, Steven Laureys, Geoffrey S. F. Ling, Risa Nakase-Richardson, Ronald T. Seel, Stuart Yablon, Thomas S. D. Getchius, Gary S. Gronseth, and Melissa J. Armstrong. "Practice Guideline Update Recommendations Summary: Disorders of Consciousness: Report of the Guideline Development, Dissemination, and Implementation Subcommittee of the American Academy of Neurology; the American Congress of Rehabilitation Medicine; and the National Institute on Disability, Independent Living, and Rehabilitation Research." *Archives of Physical Medicine and Rehabilitation* 99, no. 9 (2018): 1699–1709.

Gillett, Grant. "Consciousness, the Brain and What Matters." *Bioethics* 4, no. 3 (1990): 181–198.

Godfrey-Smith, Peter. *Metazoa: Animal Life and the Birth of the Mind*. New York: Farrar, Straus and Giroux, 2020.

Gosseries, Olivia, Marie-Aurélie Bruno, Camille Chatelle, Audrey Vanhaudenhuyse, Caroline Schnakers, Andrea Soddu, and Steven Laureys. "Disorders of Consciousness: What's in a Name?" *NeuroRehabilitation* 28, no. 1 (2011): 3–14.

Gould, Helen, Syed S. Hashmi, Victoria F. Wagner, Katie Stoll, Kathryn Ostermaier, and Jennifer Czerwinski. "Examining Genetic Counselors' Implicit Attitudes Toward Disability." *Journal of Genetic Counseling* 28, no. 6 (2019): 1098–1106.

Gray, Kurt, T. Anne Knickman, and Daniel M. Wegner. "More Dead Than Dead: Perceptions of Persons in the Persistent Vegetative State." *Cognition* 121, no. 2 (2011): 275–280.

Green, Carmen R., Karen O. Anderson, Tamara A. Baker, Lisa C. Campbell, Sheila Decker, Roger B. Fillingim, Donna A. Kaloukalani, Kathryn E. Lasch, Cynthia Myers, and Raymond C. Tait. "The Unequal Burden of Pain: Confronting Racial and Ethnic Disparities in Pain." *Pain Medicine* 4, no. 3 (2003): 277–294.

Habib, Abdella M., Andrei L. Okorokov, Matthew N. Hill, Jose T. Bras, Man-Cheung Lee, Shengnan Li, Samuel J. Gossage, Marie van Drimmelen, Maria Morena, and Henry Houlden. "Microdeletion in a FAAH Pseudogene Identified in a Patient with High Anandamide Concentrations and Pain Insensitivity." *British Journal of Anaesthesia* 123, no. 2 (2019): e249–e253.

Hale, Benjamin. "Moral Considerability: Deontological, Not Metaphysical." *Ethics and the Environment* 16, no. 2 (2011): 37–62.

Hall, Richard J., and Charles R. Johnson. "The Epistemic Duty to Seek More Evidence." *American Philosophical Quarterly* 35, no. 2 (1998): 129–139.

Hansen, Gregory, and Ari R. Joffe. "Confounding Brain Stem Function During Pediatric Brain Death Determination: Two Case Reports." *Journal of Child Neurology* 32, no. 7 (2017): 676–679.

Hardcastle, Valerie Gray. "Minimally Conscious States and Pain." In *Finding Consciousness: The Neuroscience, Ethics, and Law of Severe Brain Damage*, edited by Walter Sinnott-Armstrong, 207–225. Oxford: Oxford University Press, 2016.

Harrison, Peter. "Descartes on Animals." *The Philosophical Quarterly* 42, no. 167 (1992): 219–227.

Heine, Lizette, Steven Laureys, and Caroline Schnakers. "Behavioral Responsiveness in Patients with Disorders of Consciousness." In *Brain Function and Responsiveness in Disorders of Consciousness*, edited by Martin M. Monti and Walter G. Sannita, 25–36. Cham: Springer, 2016.

Hemphill, J. Claude, and Douglas B. White. "Clinical Nihilism in Neuroemergencies." *Emergency Medicine Clinics of North America* 27, no. 1 (2009): 27–37.

Hickson, Melissa. "Recording of Melissa Hickson and St. David's Doctor," 2020. YouTube video, https://www.youtube.com/watch?time_continue=314&v=jq-_gtjnzZg&feature=emb_logo.

High, Dallas M. "Who Will Make Health Care Decisions for Me When I Can't?" *Journal of Aging and Health* 2, no. 3 (1990): 291–309.

Holland, Stephen, Celia Kitzinger, and Jenny Kitzinger. "Death, Treatment Decisions and the Permanent Vegetative State: Evidence from Families and Experts." *Medicine, Health Care and Philosophy* 17, no. 3 (2014): 413–423.

Horta, Oscar. "The Scope of the Argument from Species Overlap." *Journal of Applied Philosophy* 31, no. 2 (2014): 142–154.

Hume, David. *A Treatise of Human Nature,* 2nd ed. Oxford, UK: Oxford University Press, 1739.

Huxley, Thomas Henry. *Lessons in Elementary Physiology.* New York: Macmillan and Company, 1890.

In re Quinlan. 1976. 355 A.2d 647, 70 N.J. 10, 70 New Jersey 10 (1976).

In re Schiavo. 2000. (Fla. Cir. Ct. Pinellas County, February 11, 2000).

In re Young. 2020. No. 15-14-GA (Fla. Cir. Ct. Liberty County, June 11, 2020).

Ingalls, Theodore H. "Pathogenesis of Mongolism." *American Journal of Diseases of Children* 73, no. 3 (1947): 279–292.

Izzy, Saef, Rebecca Compton, Raphael Carandang, Wiley Hall, and Susanne Muehlschlegel. "Self-fulfilling Prophecies Through Withdrawal of Care: Do They Exist in Traumatic Brain Injury, Too?" *Neurocritical Care* 19, no. 3 (2013): 347–363.

Jackson, Elizabeth. "What's Epistemic About Epistemic Paternalism?" In *Essays in Epistemic Autonomy,* edited by Jonathan Matheson and Kirk Lougheed, 132–150. New York: Routledge, 2021.

Jackson, Emily. "The Minimally Conscious State and Treatment Withdrawal: W v M." *Journal of Medical Ethics* 39, no. 9 (2013): 559–561.

James, William. "The Will to Believe." In *The Will to Believe: And Other Essays in Popular Philosophy,* edited by William James, 1–31. Cambridge, UK: Cambridge University Press, 2014.

Jenkins, R. L. "Etiology of Mongolism." *American Journal of Diseases of Children* 45, no. 3 (1933): 506–519.

Jennett, Bryan. "Letting Vegetative Patients Die." *BMJ: British Medical Journal* 305, no. 6865 (1992): 1305.

Jennett, Bryan, and Clare Dyer. "Persistent Vegetative State and the Right to Die: The United States and Britain." *BMJ: British Medical Journal* 302, no. 6787 (1991): 1256.

Jennett, Bryan, and Fred Plum. "Persistent Vegetative State after Brain Damage: A Syndrome in Search of a Name." *The Lancet* 299, no. 7753 (1972): 734–737.

Johnson, Harriet McBryde. "Not Dead at All: Why Congress Was Right to Stick up for Terri Schiavo." *Slate*, March 23, 2005.

Johnson, L. Syd M. "Can They Suffer? The Ethical Priority of Quality of Life Research in Disorders of Consciousness." *Bioethica Forum* 6, no. 4 (2013): 129–136.

Johnson, L. Syd M. "Withholding Care from Vegetative Patients: The Social and Financial Costs." *Bioethics Forum*, July 2, 2010, https://www.thehastingscenter.org/withholding-care-from-vegetative-patients-financial-savings-and-social-costs/.

Johnson, L. Syd M. "The Right to Die in the Minimally Conscious State." *Journal of Medical Ethics* 37, no. 3 (2011): 175–178.

Johnson, L. Syd M. "The Case for Reasonable Accommodation of Conscientious Objections to Declarations of Brain Death." *Journal of Bioethical Inquiry* 13, no. 1 (2016a): 105–115.

Johnson, L. Syd M. "Moving Beyond End of Life: The Ethics of Disorders of Consciousness in an Age of Discovery and Uncertainty." In *Brain Function and Responsiveness in Disorders of Consciousness*, edited by Martin M. Monti and Walter G. Sannita, 185–194. Cham: Springer, 2016b.

Johnson, L. Syd M. "Death by Neurological Criteria: Expert Definitions and Lay Misgivings." *QJM: An International Journal of Medicine* 110, no. 5 (2017a): 267–270.

Johnson, L. Syd M. "Known Unknowns: Diagnosis and Prognosis in Disorders of Consciousness." *AJOB Neuroscience* 8, no. 3 (2017b): 145–146.

Johnson, L. Syd M. 2020a. "Prioritizing Justice in Ventilator Allocation." *Journal of Medical Ethics Blog*, April 15, 2020, https://blogs.bmj.com/medical-ethics/2020/04/15/prioritizing-justice-in-ventilator-allocation/.

Johnson, L. Syd M. "The Trouble with Animal Models in Brain Research." In *Neuroethics and Nonhuman Animals*, edited by L. Syd M Johnson, Andrew Fenton, and Adam Shriver, 271–286. Cham: Springer, 2020b.

Johnson, L. Syd M, and Kathy L. Cerminara. "All Things Considered: Surrogate Decision-Making on Behalf of Patients in the Minimally Conscious State." *Clinical Ethics* 15, no. 3 (2020): 111–119.

Johnson, L. Syd M, and Christos Lazaridis. "The Sources of Uncertainty in Disorders of Consciousness." *AJOB Neuroscience* 9, no. 2 (2018): 76–82.

Johnson, Mary. "Terri Schiavo: A Disability Rights Case." *Death Studies* 30, no. 2 (2006): 163–176.

Jonsen, Albert R. "The Birth of Bioethics." *The Hastings Center Report* 23, no. 6 (1993): S1–S4.

Joyce, James. *Finnegans Wake*. New York: Penguin Books, 1939.

Kalanithi, Paul. 2014. "How Long Have I Got Left?" *The New York Times*, January 24, 2014, SR:9, https://www.nytimes.com/2014/01/25/opinion/sunday/how-long-have-i-got-left.html.

Kaposy, Chris. "A Disability Critique of the New Prenatal Test for Down Syndrome." *Kennedy Institute of Ethics Journal* 23, no. 4 (2013): 299–324.

Kaposy, Chris. *Choosing Down Syndrome: Ethics and New Prenatal Testing Technologies.* Cambridge, MA: MIT Press, 2018.

Katz, Douglas I., Meg Polyak, Daniel Coughlan, Meliné Nichols, and Alexis Roche. "Natural History of Recovery from Brain Injury after Prolonged Disorders of Consciousness: Outcome of Patients Admitted to Inpatient Rehabilitation with 1–4 Year Follow-up." *Progress in Brain Research* 177 (2009): 73–88.

Kaufmann, Mark A., Barbara Buchmann, Daniel Scheidegger, Otmar Gratzl, and Ernst W. Radü. "Severe Head Injury: Should Expected Outcome Influence Resuscitation and First-Day Decisions?" *Resuscitation* 23, no. 3 (1992): 199–206.

Kinney, Hannah C., Julius Korein, Ashok Panigrahy, Pieter Dikkes, and Robert Goode. "Neuropathological Findings in the Brain of Karen Ann Quinlan—The Role of the Thalamus in the Persistent Vegetative State." *The New England Journal of Medicine* 330, no. 21 (1994): 1469–1475.

Kitzinger, Celia, and Jenny Kitzinger. "'This In-Between': How Families Talk about Death in Relation to Severe Brain Injury and Disorders of Consciousness." In *The Social Construction of Death*, edited by Leen Van Brussel and Nico Carpentier, 239–258. London, UK: Palgrave Macmillan, 2014.

Kitzinger, Jenny, and Celia Kitzinger. "The 'Window of Opportunity' for Death after Severe Brain Injury: Family Experiences." *Sociology of Health & Illness* 35, no. 7 (2013): 1095–1112.

Klein, Colin. "Consciousness, Intention, and Command-Following in the Vegetative State." *British Journal for the Philosophy of Science* 68, no. 1 (2015): 27–54.

Koch, Christof. *The Quest for Consciousness: A Neurobiological Approach.* Englewood, CO: Roberts & Company, 2004.

Kon, Alexander A., Eric K. Shepard, Nneka O. Sederstrom, Sandra M. Swoboda, Mary Faith Marshall, Barbara Birriel, and Fred Rincon. "Defining Futile and Potentially Inappropriate Interventions: A Policy Statement From the Society of Critical Care Medicine Ethics Committee." *Critical Care Medicine* 44, no. 9 (2016): 1769–1774.

Kuehlmeyer, Katja, Corinna Klingler, Eric Racine, and Ralf J. Jox. "Single Case Reports on Late Recovery from Chronic Disorders of Consciousness: A Systematic Review and Ethical Appraisal." *Bioethica Forum* 6 (2013): 137–149.

Latorre, Julius Gene S., Elena B. Schmidt, and David M. Greer. "Another Pitfall in Brain Death Diagnosis: Return of Cerebral Function after Determination of Brain Death by Both Clinical and Radionuclide Cerebral Perfusion Imaging." *Neurocritical Care* 32 (2020): 899–905.

Laureys, Steven. "The Neural Correlate of (Un)awareness: Lessons from the Vegetative State." *Trends in Cognitive Sciences* 9, no. 12 (2005): 556–559.

Laureys, Steven, Gastone G. Celesia, Francois Cohadon, Jan Lavrijsen, José León-Carrión, Walter G. Sannita, Leon Sazbon, Erich Schmutzhard, Klaus R. von Wild, and Adam Zeman. "Unresponsive Wakefulness Syndrome: A New Name for the Vegetative State or Apallic Syndrome." *BMC Medicine* 8, no. 1 (2010): 68.

Lavery, James V. "'Wicked Problems', Community Engagement and the Need for an Implementation Science for Research Ethics." *Journal of Medical Ethics* 44, no. 3 (2018): 163–164.

Lazaridis, Christos. "Withdrawal of Life-Sustaining Treatments in Perceived Devastating Brain Injury: The Key Role of Uncertainty." *Neurocritical Care* 30, no. 1 (2019): 33–41.

Lazaridis, Christos, Masoom Desai, and L. Syd M Johnson. "Communication and Well-Being Considerations in Disorders of Consciousness." *Neurocritical Care* 34 (2021): 701–703, https://doi.org/10.1007/s12028-020-01175-z.

Levy, Neil. "What Difference Does Consciousness Make?" *Monash Bioethics Review* 28, no. 2 (2009): 13–25.

Levy, Neil, and Julian Savulescu. "Moral Significance of Phenomenal Consciousness." *Progress in Brain Research* 177 (2009): 361–370.

Locke, John. *An Essay Concerning Human Understanding.* Oxford, UK: Oxford University Press. Original edition, 1689.

Lulé, Dorothée, Claudia Zickler, S Häcker, Marie-Aurelie Bruno, Athena Demertzi, Frederic Pellas, Steven Laureys, and A Kübler. "Life Can Be Worth Living in Locked-in Syndrome." *Progress in Brain Research* 177 (2009): 339–351.

Lunau, Kate. 2015. "The Story Behind a Vegetative Patient's Shocking Recovery." *Maclean's*, December 31, 2015.

Macniven, J. A., R. Poz, K. Bainbridge, F. Gracey, and B. A. Wilson. "Emotional Adjustment Following Cognitive Recovery from 'Persistent Vegetative State': Psychological and Personal Perspectives." *Brain Injury* 17, no. 6 (2003): 525–533.

Mayer, Stephan A., and Sharon B. Kossoff. "Withdrawal of Life Support in the Neurological Intensive Care Unit." *Neurology* 52, no. 8 (1999): 1602–1609.

McMahan, Jeff. "The Metaphysics of Brain Death." *Bioethics* 9, no. 2 (1995): 91–126.

McMahan, Jeff. "Brain Death, Cortical Death, and Persistent Vegetative State." In *A Companion to Bioethics,* edited by Helga Kuhse and Peter Singer, 250–260. Oxford, UK: Blackwell, 1998.

Menon, David K., A. M. Owen, S. J. Boniface, and J. D. Pickard. "Cortical Processing in Persistent Vegetative State." *The Lancet* 352, no. 9134 (1998): 1148–1149.

Mill, John Stuart. *Utilitarianism.* New York: Bobbs-Merrill Company, 1861.

Mirzaei, Komeil, Alireza Milanifar, and Fariba Asghari. "Patients' Perspectives of the Substitute Decision Maker: Who Makes Better Decisions?" *Journal of Medical Ethics* 37, no. 9 (2011): 523–525.

Monti, Martin M. "Cognition in the Vegetative State." *Annual Review of Clinical Psychology* 8 (2012): 431–454.

Monti, Martin M. "Disorders of Consciousness." In *Emerging Trends in the Social and Behavioral Sciences* edited by Robert Scott and Stephan Kosslyn, 1–13. Hoboken: John Wiley & Sons, 2015.

Monti, Martin M., and Adrian M. Owen. "Behavior in the Brain." *Journal of Psychophysiology* 24 (2010): 76–82.

Monti, Martin M., Audrey Vanhaudenhuyse, Martin R. Coleman, Melanie Boly, John D. Pickard, Luaba Tshibanda, Adrian M. Owen, and Steven Laureys. "Willful Modulation of Brain Activity in Disorders of Consciousness." *The New England Journal of Medicine* 362, no. 7 (2010): 579–589.

Multi-Society Task Force on PVS. "Medical Aspects of the Persistent Vegetative State: Prognosis for Recovery." *The New England Journal of Medicine* 330, no. 22 (1994): 1572–1579.

Murphy, Heather. "At 71, She's Never Felt Pain or Anxiety. Now Scientists Know Why." *The New York Times,* March 28, 2019, A7.

Naccache, Lionel. "Minimally Conscious State or Cortically Mediated State?" *Brain* 141, no. 4 (2017): 949–960.

Naci, Lorina, Rhodri Cusack, Mimma Anello, and Adrian M. Owen. "A Common Neural Code for Similar Conscious Experiences in Different Individuals." *Proceedings of the National Academy of Sciences* 111, no. 39 (2014): 14277–14282.

Nakase-Richardson, Risa, John Whyte, Joseph T. Giacino, Shital Pavawalla, Scott D. Barnett, Stuart A. Yablon, Mark Sherer, Kathleen Kalmar, Flora M. Hammond, and Brian Greenwald. "Longitudinal Outcome of Patients with Disordered Consciousness in the NIDRR TBI Model Systems Programs." *Journal of Neurotrauma* 29, no. 1 (2012): 59–65.

Nardini, Marko, Rachael Bedford, and Denis Mareschal. "Fusion of Visual Cues Is Not Mandatory in Children." *Proceedings of the National Academy of Sciences* 107, no. 39 (2010): 17041–17046.

National Disability Alliance Steering Committee. "Statement from the National Disability Leadership Alliance on Racism and Bias Within the Disability Community and Movement," 2020, http://www.disabilityleadership.org/news/statement-from-the-national-disability-leadership-alliance-on-racism-and-bias-within-the-disability-community-and-movement/.

Natoli, Jaime L., Deborah L. Ackerman, Suzanne McDermott, and Janice G. Edwards. "Prenatal Diagnosis of Down Syndrome: A Systematic Review of Termination Rates (1995–2011)." *Prenatal Diagnosis* 32, no. 2 (2012): 142–153.

Noonan, John T. *The Morality of Abortion: Legal and Historical Perspectives* Cambridge, US: Harvard University Press, 1971.

Norcross, Alastair. "Puppies, Pigs, and People: Eating Meat and Marginal Cases." *Philosophical Perspectives* 18 (2004): 229–245.

Ong, Matthew. "Amy Reed, Physician and Patient Who "Moved Mountains" to End Widespread Use of Power Morcellation, Dies at 44." *The Cancer Letter*, May 26, 2017, https://cancerletter.com/articles/20170526_1/.

Orentlicher, David. "The Illusion of Patient Choice in End-of-Life Decisions." *JAMA* 267, no. 15 (1992): 2101–2104.

Ouellette, Alicia. "When Vitalism Is Dead Wrong: The Discrimination Against and Torture of Incompetent Patients by Compulsory Life-Sustaining Treatment." *Indiana Law Journal* 79 (2004): 1–55.

Ouellette, Alicia. "Disability and the End of Life." *Oregon Law Review* 85, no. 123 (2006): 123–182.

Overbeek, Berno U. H., Henk J. Eilander, Jan C. M. Lavrijsen, and Raymond T. C. M. Koopmans. "Are Visual Functions Diagnostic Signs of the Minimally Conscious State? An Integrative Review." *Journal of Neurology* 265, no. 9 (2018): 1957–1975.

Owen, Adrian M., Martin R. Coleman, Melanie Boly, Matthew H. Davis, Steven Laureys, and John D. Pickard. "Detecting Awareness in the Vegetative State." *Science* 313, no. 5792 (2006): 1402.

Parens, Erik, and Adrienne Asch. *Prenatal Testing and Disability Rights*. Washington, DC: Georgetown University Press, 2000.

Patterson, David, and Alberto C. S. Costa. "Down Syndrome and Genetics—A Case of Linked Histories." *Nature Reviews Genetics* 6, no. 2 (2005): 137–147.

Pistorius, Martin. *Ghost Boy: The Miraculous Escape of a Misdiagnosed Boy Trapped Inside His Own Body*. Nashville, TN: Thomas Nelson, 2013.

Plato. "Philebus." In *Plato: Complete Works*, edited by John H. Cooper, 398–456. Indianapolis: Hackett, 1997.

Pohlhaus, Gaile, Jr. "Relational Knowing and Epistemic Injustice: Toward a Theory of Willful Hermeneutical Ignorance." *Hypatia* 27, no. 4 (2012): 715–735.

Poldrack, Russell A. "Inferring Mental States from Neuroimaging Data: From Reverse Inference to Large-Scale Decoding." *Neuron* 72, no. 5 (2011): 692–697.

Popat, Shreeya, and William Winslade. "While You Were Sleepwalking: Science and Neurobiology of Sleep Disorders & the Enigma of Legal Responsibility of Violence During Parasomnia." *Neuroethics* 8, no. 2 (2015): 203–214.

Pound, Pandora, and Christine J. Nicol. "Retrospective Harm Benefit Analysis of Pre-clinical Animal Research for Six Treatment Interventions." *PLOS One* 13, no. 3 (2018): e0193758.

Pound, Pandora, and Merel Ritskes-Hoitinga. "Is It Possible to Overcome Issues of External Validity in Preclinical Animal Research? Why Most

Animal Models Are Bound to Fail." *Journal of Translational Medicine* 16, no. 1 (2018): 1–8.

President's Council on Bioethics. *Controversies in the Determination of Death: A White Paper of the President's Council on Bioethics.* Washington, DC: U.S. Government Printing Office, 2008.

Provencio, J. Javier, J. Claude Hemphill, Jan Claassen, Brian L. Edlow, Raimund Helbok, Paul M. Vespa, Michael N. Diringer, Len Polizzotto, Lori Shutter, and Jose I. Suarez. "The Curing Coma Campaign: Framing Initial Scientific Challenges—Proceedings of the First Curing Coma Campaign Scientific Advisory Council Meeting." *Neurocritical Care* 33 (2020): 1–12.

Rabinstein, Alejandro A., and J. Claude Hemphill. "Prognosticating after Severe Acute Brain Disease: Science, Art, and Biases." *Neurology* 74, no. 14 (2010): 1086–1087.

Rachels, James. "Drawing Lines." In *Animal Rights: Current Debates and New Directions,* edited by Cass R. Sunstein and Martha C. Nussbaum, 162–174. Oxford, UK: Oxford University Press, 2004.

Rahdert, George K., Max Lapertosa, Kenneth M. Walden, and Aliza Kaliski. "Brief of Amici Curiae Not Dead Yet et al., *Jeb Bush v. Michael Schiavo.*" *Issues in Law & Medicine* 20, no. 2 (2004): 171.

Rapp, Emily. *The Still Point of the Turning World.* New York: Penguin Books, 2014.

Ravelingien, An, Freddy Mortier, Eric Mortier, Ilse Kerremans, and Johan Braeckman. "Proceeding with Clinical Trials of Animal to Human Organ Transplantation: A Way out of the Dilemma." *Journal of Medical Ethics* 30, no. 1 (2004): 92–98.

Redpath, S. J., W. Huw Williams, D. Hanna, M. A. Linden, P. Yates, and Anthony Harris. "Healthcare Professionals' Attitudes Towards Traumatic Brain Injury (TBI): The Influence of Profession, Experience, Aetiology and Blame on Prejudice Towards Survivors of Brain Injury." *Brain Injury* 24, no. 6 (2010): 802–811.

Regan, Tom. *The Case for Animal Rights.* Berkeley: University of California Press, 2004.

Reynolds, Joel Michael. ""I'd Rather Be Dead Than Disabled"—The Ableist Conflation and the Meanings of Disability." *Review of Communication* 17, no. 3 (2017): 149–163.

Rich, Ben A. "Prospective Autonomy and Critical Interests: A Narrative Defense of the Moral Authority of Advance Directives." *Cambridge Quarterly of Healthcare Ethics* 6, no. 2 (1997): 138–147.

Rittel, Horst W. J., and Melvin M. Webber. "Dilemmas in a General Theory of Planning." *Policy Sciences* 4, no. 2 (1973): 155–169.

Robbins, William. "Parents Fight for Right To Let a Daughter Die." *The New York Times,* November 27, 1989, B, https://www.nytimes.com/1989/11/27/us/parents-fight-for-right-to-let-a-daughter-die.html.

Rocker, Graeme, Deborah Cook, Peter Sjokvist, Bruce Weaver, Simon Finfer, Ellen McDonald, John Marshall, et al. "Clinician Predictions of Intensive Care Unit Mortality." *Critical Care Medicine* 32, no. 5 (2004): 1149–1154.

Rosenbaum, R. Shayna, Stefan Köhler, Daniel L. Schacter, Morris Moscovitch, Robyn Westmacott, Sandra E. Black, Fuqiang Gao, and Endel Tulving. "The Case of K.C.: Contributions of a Memory-Impaired Person to Memory Theory." *Neuropsychologia* 43, no.7 (2005): 989–1021.

Rowlands, Mark. *Can Animals Be Moral?* Oxford, UK: Oxford University Press, 2012.

Royal College of Physicians. "Criteria for the Diagnosis of Brain Stem Death. Review by a Working Group Convened by the Royal College of Physicians and Endorsed by the Conference of Medical Royal Colleges and Their Faculties in the United Kingdom." *Journal of the Royal College of Physicians of London* 29, no. 5 (1995): 381–382.

Rudner, Richard. "The Scientist Qua Scientist Makes Value Judgments." *Philosophy of Science* 20, no. 1 (1953): 1–6.

Sachs, Benjamin. "The Status of Moral Status." *Pacific Philosophical Quarterly* 92, no. 1 (2011): 87–104.

Schiff, Nicholas D. "Cognitive Motor Dissociation Following Severe Brain Injuries." *JAMA Neurology* 72, no. 12 (2015): 1413–1415.

Schloendorff v. New York Hospital, 211 N.Y. 125, 105 N.E. 92 (N.Y. 1914).

Schnakers, Caroline, Camille Chatelle, Athina Demertzi, Steve Majerus, and Steven Laureys. "What About Pain in Disorders of Consciousness?" *The AAPS Journal* 14, no. 3 (2012): 437–444.

Schnakers, Caroline, Camille Chatelle, Audrey Vanhaudenhuyse, Steve Majerus, Didier Ledoux, Melanie Boly, Marie-Aurélie Bruno, Pierre Boveroux, Athena Demertzi, and Gustave Moonen. "The Nociception Coma Scale: A New Tool to Assess Nociception in Disorders of Consciousness." *Pain* 148, no. 2 (2010): 215–219.

Schnakers, Caroline, Audrey Vanhaudenhuyse, Joseph Giacino, Manfredi Ventura, Melanie Boly, Steve Majerus, Gustave Moonen, and Steven Laureys. "Diagnostic Accuracy of the Vegetative and Minimally Conscious State: Clinical Consensus Versus Standardized Neurobehavioral Assessment." *BMC Neurology* 9, no. 35 (2009).

Schnakers, Caroline, and Nathan D Zasler. "Pain Assessment and Management in Disorders of Consciousness." *Current Opinion in Neurology* 20, no. 6 (2007): 620–626.

Schwartz, Carolyn E., Elena M. Andresen, Margaret A. Nosek, and Gloria L. Krahn. "Response Shift Theory: Important Implications for Measuring Quality of Life in People with Disability." *Archives of Physical Medicine and Rehabilitation* 88, no. 4 (2009): 529–536.

Seth, Anil. "Explanatory Correlates of Consciousness: Theoretical and Computational Challenges." *Cognitive Computation* 1 (2009): 50–63.

Shakespeare, Tom. "The Social Model of Disability." In *The Disability Studies Reader*, edited by Lennard J. Davis, 197–204. London, UK: Routledge, 2006.

Shapiro, Joseph. "One Man's COVID-19 Death Raises the Worst Fears of Many People with Disabilities." Washington, DC: National Public Radio, 2020, https://www.npr.org/2020/07/31/896882268/one-mans-covid-19-death-raises-the-worst-fears-of-many-people-with-disabilities.

Shepherd, Joshua. *Consciousness and Moral Status*. New York: Routledge, 2018.

Sherry, Mark. *If I Only Had a Brain: Deconstructing Brain Injury*. New York: Routledge, 2013.

Shewmon, D. Alan. "Chronic Brain Death: Meta-analysis and Conceptual Consequences." *Neurology* 51, no. 6 (1998): 1538–1545.

Shewmon, D. Alan. "A Critical Analysis of Conceptual Domains of the Vegetative State: Sorting Fact from Fancy." *NeuroRehabilitation* 19, no. 4 (2004): 343–347.

Shewmon, D. Alan. "False-Positive Diagnosis of Brain Death Following the Pediatric Guidelines: Case Report and Discussion." *Journal of Child Neurology* 32, no. 14 (2017): 1104–1117.

Shewmon, D. Alan. "The Case of Jahi McMath: A Neurologist's View." *Hastings Center Report* 48, no. S4 (2018): S74–S76.

Smith, Alexander K., Douglas B. White, and Robert M. Arnold. "Uncertainty: The Other Side of Prognosis." *The New England Journal of Medicine* 368, no. 26 (2013): 2448–2450.

Specker Sullivan, Laura. "Pure Experience and Disorders of Consciousness." *AJOB Neuroscience* 9, no. 2 (2018): 107–114.

Spohn, Stephen. @stevenspohn: Twitter, 2020, https://twitter.com/stevenspohn/status/1277681028166037504.

Sprung, C. L., S. L. Cohen, P. Sjokvist, et al. "End-of-life Practices in European Intensive Care Units: The Ethicus Study." *JAMA* 290, no. 6 (2003): 790–797.

Steppacher, Inga, Michael Kaps, and Johanna Kissler. "Will Time Heal? A Long-Term Follow-up of Severe Disorders of Consciousness." *Annals of Clinical and Translational Neurology* 1, no. 6 (2014): 401–408.

Steppacher, Inga, Michael Kaps, and Johanna Kissler. "Against the Odds: A Case Study of Recovery from Coma after Devastating Prognosis." *Annals of Clinical and Translational Neurology* 3, no. 1 (2016): 61–65.

Steppacher, Inga, and Johanna Kissler. "The Living Dead? Perception of Persons in the Unresponsive Wakefulness Syndrome in Germany Compared to the USA." *BMC Psychology* 6, no. 1 (2018): 1–12.

Stramondo, Joseph. "Disabled by Design: Justifying and Limiting Parental Authority to Choose Future Children with Pre-implantation Genetic Diagnosis." *Kennedy Institute of Ethics Journal* 27, no. 4 (2017): 475–500.

Sullivan, Mark D. "The Illusion of Patient Choice in End-of-Life Decisions." *The American Journal of Geriatric Psychiatry* 10, no. 4 (2002): 365–372.

Tangwa, Godfrey B. "The Traditional African Perception of a Person: Some Implications for Bioethics." *Hastings Center Report* 30, no. 5 (2000): 39–43.

Tavalaro, Julia, and Richard Tayson. *Look Up for Yes*. Tokyo: Kodansha International, 1997.

Thomas, Lewis. "The Technology of Medicine." *The New England Journal of Medicine* 285, no. 24 (1971): 1366–1368.

Tononi, Giulio, Melanie Boly, Marcello Massimini, and Christof Koch. "Integrated Information Theory: From Consciousness to Its Physical Substrate." *Nature Reviews Neuroscience* 17, no. 7 (2016): 450–461.

Tooley, Michael. "Abortion and Infanticide." *Philosophy & Public Affairs* 2, no. 1 (1972): 37–65.

Turgeon, Alexis F., François Lauzier, Jean-François Simard, Damon C. Scales, Karen E. A. Burns, Lynne Moore, David A. Zygun, Francis Bernard, Maureen O. Meade, and Tran Cong Dung. "Mortality Associated with Withdrawal of Life-Sustaining Therapy for Patients with Severe Traumatic Brain Injury: A Canadian Multicentre Cohort Study." *Canadian Medical Association Journal* 183, no. 14 (2011): 1581–1588.

van Erp, Willemijn S., Anoek M. L. Aben, Jan C. M. Lavrijsen, Pieter E. Vos, Steven Laureys, and Raymond T. C. M. Koopmans. "Unexpected Emergence from the Vegetative State: Delayed Discovery Rather Than Late Recovery of Consciousness." *Journal of Neurology* 266, no. 12 (2019): 3144–3149.

van Erp, Willemijn S., Jan C. M. Lavrijsen, Pieter E. Vos, Hans Bor, Steven Laureys, and Raymond T. C. M. Koopmans. "The Vegetative State: Prevalence, Misdiagnosis, and Treatment Limitations." *Journal of the American Medical Directors Association* 16, no. 1 (2015): 85e9–85e14.

van Gulick, Robert. "Consciousness." In *Stanford Encyclopedia of Philosophy*, edited by Edward N. Zalta. Stanford, CA: Stanford University, 2018. https://plato.stanford.edu/entries/consciousness/

VanPuymbrouck, Laura, Carli Friedman, and Heather Feldner. "Explicit and Implicit Disability Attitudes of Healthcare Providers." *Rehabilitation Psychology* 65, no. 2 (2020): 101–112.

Veatch, Robert M. "The Death of Whole-Brain Death: The Plague of the Disaggregators, Somaticists, and Mentalists." *Journal of Medicine and Philosophy* 30, no. 4 (2005): 353–378.

Verkade, Martijn A., Jelle L. Epker, Mariska D. Nieuwenhoff, Jan Bakker, and Erwin J. O. Kompanje. "Withdrawal of Life-Sustaining Treatment in a Mixed Intensive Care Unit: Most Common in Patients with Catastropic Brain Injury." *Neurocritical Care* 16, no. 1 (2012): 130–135.

Voss, Henning U., Aziz M. Uluç, Jonathan P. Dyke, Richard Watts, Erik J. Kobylarz, Bruce D. McCandliss, Linda A. Heier, Bradley J. Beattie, Klaus A. Hamacher, and Shankar Vallabhajosula. "Possible Axonal Regrowth in Late Recovery from the Minimally Conscious State." *The Journal of Clinical Investigation* 116, no. 7 (2006): 2005–2011.

W v M [2011] EWHC 2443 (Fam): Court of Protection.

Wager, Tor D., Lauren Y. Atlas, Martin A. Lindquist, Mathieu Roy, Choong-Wan Woo, and Ethan Kross. "An fMRI-Based Neurologic Signature of Physical Pain." *The New England Journal of Medicine* 368, no. 15 (2013): 1388–1397.

Warren, Mary Anne. "On the Moral and Legal Status of Abortion." *The Monist* 57, no. 1 (1973): 43–61.

Warren, Mary Anne. *Moral Status: Obligations to Persons and Other Living Things*. Oxford, UK: Clarendon Press, 1997.

Weinstein, Milton C., George Torrance, and Alistair McGuire. "QALYs: The Basics." *Value in Health* 12 (2009): S5–S9.

Wendell, Susan. "Unhealthy Disabled: Treating Chronic Illnesses as Disabilities." *Hypatia* 16, no. 4 (2001): 17–33.

Whyte, Kyle Powys, and Paul B. Thompson. "Ideas for How to Take Wicked Problems Seriously." *Journal of Agricultural and Environmental Ethics* 25, no. 4 (2012): 441–445.

Wilkinson, D., P. Thiele, A. Watkins, and L. De Crespigny. "Fatally Flawed? A Review and Ethical Analysis of Lethal Congenital Malformations." *BJOG: An International Journal of Obstetrics & Gynaecology* 119, no. 11 (2012): 1302–1308.

Wilkinson, Dominic. "The Window of Opportunity for Treatment Withdrawal." *Archives of Pediatrics & Adolescent Medicine* 165, no. 3 (2011): 211–215.

Wilkinson, Dominic, and Julian Savulescu. "Is It Better to be Minimally Conscious Than Vegetative?" *Journal of Medical Ethics* 39, no. 9 (2013): 557–558.

Willems, Michelle, Davide Sattin, Ad Vingerhoets, and Matilde Leonardi. "Longitudinal Changes in Functioning and Disability in Patients with Disorders of Consciousness: The Importance of Environmental Factors." *International Journal of Environmental Research and Public Health* 12, no. 4 (2015): 3707–3730.

Williams, Bernard. *Ethics and the Limits of Philosophy*. London, UK: Routledge, 2011.

Wilson, Barbara A., Fergus Gracey, and Kate Bainbridge. "Cognitive Recovery from 'Persistent Vegetative State': Psychological and Personal Perspectives." *Brain Injury* 15, no. 12 (2001): 1083–1092.

Winkielman, Piotr, and Kent C. Berridge. "Unconscious Emotion." *Current Directions in Psychological Science* 13, no. 3 (2004): 120–123.

Index